THE ANTI-INFLAMMATORY DIET FOR BEGINNERS

The Step-By-Step Guide to Prevent Cancer and All Degenerative Diseases, Anti-Inflammatory Foods and Foods to Avoid. Delicious Recipes and Meal Plans to Improve Your Immune System, Live Healthy, and Be More Energetic.

CAROLE J. LAWSON

TABLE OF CONTENTS

INTRODUCTION

Thank you, and congratulations on taking the first step towards building a healthier you! Within this book, you will find a variety of methods and tips to begin improving your health and taking control of your body from the inside out.

Before we begin, I want to give a brief disclaimer: This book is not intended to replace medical advice. It is not responsible for the actions or the results of the reader. Please seek out the advice of a doctor before starting any health program. The author is not a medical doctor, and the information in this book is meant only to supplement your health decisions and actions, not dictate them. The wonders of autophagy are still being discovered as this book is being written. Please enjoy the information provided but also be wise in consuming it.

What Is Inflammation?

I am going to begin by defining the term inflammation for you before we begin delving deeper into what it is and how it can affect your body and life as a whole.

Inflammation is, in its simplest form, the body's way of using the immune system to get rid of some kind of irritant. This irritant could be a disease, a bacterium, a cut or a scrape, or any other kind of damage or threat of damage to the body. Inflammation is a natural process in the body that is in place to help keep your body working and healthy.

To you, on the outside, inflammation may seem like it is an annoying problem that your body causes you, as it feels like swelling, redness, and pain. In reality, though, it is actually a sign of your body working tirelessly to keep you healthy and remove whatever isn't supposed to be there that is making you sick. Our bodies would not be able to heal if it were not for the presence of inflammation.

A problem arises, however, when this inflammation does not go away when it is not needed anymore in the body. For example, when your wound heals or when the threat of disease is no longer present. When this happens, a person can be left with many negative side-effects, including chronic pain, or a variety of different inflammation-related diseases. We will discuss these at length in this book.

The WHO Calls Inflammation a Threat to Human Health

The World Health Organization, or The WHO, is a worldwide organization that works to study and understand diseases and other threats to human health. In 2020, The WHO stated that diseases related to chronic inflammation are the number one cause of death in the entire world. This has sparked a lot of conversation about inflammation in the body, inflammatory diseases, and how they can be prevented before they begin. The WHO also stated that the prevalence of chronic inflammatory diseases is projected to increase greatly over the next thirty years. With statistics such as these, there has never been a better time to read this book and to begin taking your health into your own hands.

What This Book Will Teach You

In this book, I will begin by helping you to understand more about inflammation, including where it comes from, why it exists, and the reasons why it often malfunctions in this day and age. After all, it was originally meant to help maintain our health, so why now is it the biggest threat to human health? We will discuss this and what you can do about it in this book. We will also look at how you can determine if you are suffering from chronic inflammation and what this may mean for you. We will then discuss several of the most common inflammatory diseases and how they come about in the body. This will help you understand how you can prevent them, especially if you have a family history of any of them. We are then going to delve deeply into something called the Anti-Inflammatory Diet, which is a new way of eating that has the potential to change your life forever. We will look at what this diet is, how it can benefit you, and what kinds of foods are included in this new way of eating. I will then share with you some recipe examples so that you can get started on this new diet right away, and I will share with you the foods that you should be eating much more of and the ones that you should avoid altogether. To finish, I will provide you with a sample meal plan to help get you started, and I will share with you several tips that will help you to stick to your new diet in the long-term so that you can continue to improve and maintain your health for the rest of your life.

We will begin the first chapter by talking about the science of inflammation, so continue reading to being learning about how inflammation works and why it has become such a challenge for so many people in 2020.

Chapter 1

The Science of Inflammation

In this chapter, we will delve into the science of inflammation so that you can begin to get a better understanding of what exactly it is and how it may be affecting your body. We will look at how it is caused and the effects that it has, before moving onto the science of how it became such a problem in our present day.

Why Is Inflammation a Problem Today?

There are a variety of things that can contribute to inflammation in a person's body. In today's world, especially, many lifestyle factors contribute to high levels of inflammation in a person's body. Below are several of the factors that can lead to chronic inflammation in the body, and which can eventually lead to inflammatory diseases, which we will look at in the next chapter.

- **Smoking**

Long-term smoking can lead to chronic inflammation in the body because of all of the chemicals that are being brought into the tissues of the body.

- **Obesity**

Obesity leads to inflammation in the body as it has negative effects on the inflammatory cells that are stored within fat deposits in the body.

- **Alcohol Use**

Alcohol use over time can lead to chronic inflammation in the intestines of the body, which then will lead to problems in the body's ability to control and adjust the levels of inflammation in the intestines afterward. Over time, this can lead to a chronic problem in the body and inflammatory diseases.

- **Chronic Stress**

According to recent statistics, nearly 40% of people reported that their levels of stress have gone up over the last year, and almost 45% said their stress had increased significantly over the past five years.

Numerous experts across the globe all agree that thinking stress is only a psychological feeling is a very dangerous misconception. They used an analogy to explain this further. Since the human stress response has evolved over the millions of years, it originally helped our ancestors identify danger and food. This is very natural; without it, humans would be trying to befriend bears rather than gathering berries from forests. There are a lot of threats back in those days that range from avoiding predators to finding food. This is completely natural, and without our stress response, we would've never made it this far. However, what isn't natural is how modern life exposes us to milder threats, but the stress we feel is constant. This is due to being overwhelmed with stimulation, juggling too many things, multitasking, and being always on the go. In simpler terms, humans were not designed to run away from predators for 10+ hours per day without any breaks. Essentially, this is what humans are doing in modern-day society.

Many experts have named the common condition of chronic stress in our society as "super stress." Humans are now being overwhelmed with numerous stressors that we almost take for granted. This includes; inadequate salaries, job dissatisfaction, being overworked, not having enough time for family and friends, lack of time outside, noise pollution, and feeling like their life has no purpose or meaning. The crazy part about all of this is that our body cannot physically differentiate the difference between being attacked by a bear and getting a bad job review. The chemical and biological response in our body is the exact same. Due to this, the body begins to get worn down due to the intensity of the stress.

When a person continuously lives with chronic stress, their emotional and behavioral actions can become ingrained within them. The wiring of their brain and body begins to change and makes them more prone to the negative effects that stress has on a person's body regardless of what's actually happening to them. Stress leads to an over-active immune system since the body cannot tell the difference between stress in the mind and stress in the body. This leads the body to initiate an immune response, which, over time, can become chronic if the stress is also chronic. Chronic stress can be so dangerous, in fact, that it can kill people due to long-term body damage in the form of heart attacks, strokes, and even cancer, all of which are diseases related to inflammation.

- **The Yo-Yo Blood Sugar Effect**

We will now discuss something known as the yo-yo blood sugar effect. This is something that happens in our bodies when we consume too much refined sugar. This is becoming a problem in today's societies as the amount of sugar we regularly consume is more than ever before. This is causing problems for people like type 2 diabetes, obesity, and heart problems. The reason that sugar causes this is the following;

When we consume regular sugar, like natural sugars found in fruits, for example, our body has to transform it through digestion into a simpler form of sugar that can travel through our blood and give us energy. It does this in a controlled way at a steady pace that is perfect for the amount of sugar we need in our bloodstream. However, when we eat sugars that are refined- like white sugar and High Fructose Corn Syrup, this sugar already comes in this simple form that is carried through the blood. This means that the body doesn't have to transform it, and it is already able to enter the bloodstream. When we eat this type, it goes directly into our blood, and this makes for a sugar overload. This is called a blood sugar spike. Our body then can't use up all of the sugar fast enough, and it starts to cause a sort of back up in the bloodstream. In order to try to deal with this, the body releases a hormone that is called insulin. Insulin is likely something you have heard of before. What insulin does it take the extra sugar in the blood and send it to be stored for later, when we need energy.

Now, this wouldn't be too terrible if it happened once in a while, but the problem is that when refined sugar is consumed over and over again, this begins to become a bigger problem. When our body receives a quick and large insulin spike, it lowers blood sugar by a larger amount than it normally would after a regular meal, in order to counter this large spike and prepare itself for a possible overload of sugar. It does this because its main job in the body is to maintain a regular level of blood sugar. After this blood sugar drops the high levels of responsive insulin cause, we will have a middle to low blood sugar level. When we then eat something sugary again, our blood sugar will spike once again, and the body will react accordingly once again. This effect is called the yo-yo blood sugar effect.

The yo-yo blood sugar effect is hard on our cells and our organs, as it makes them work overtime, trying to compensate for the high levels of refined sugar that we are putting into it. This puts stress on our organs, cells, and body systems and eventually can make them weaker. The other part of the body that sugar negatively affects is the brain. Since the rest of the body is working so hard to accommodate the spikes and dips in blood sugar levels, the brain still needs fuel. While it would usually get fuel from the food, the body is working hard to process; if the body is processing refined sugars, there are no nutrients to send to the brain. This means that it must be fed some other way, and this is done through stored nutrients from other meals. If there are no stored nutrients, though, there is no fuel for the brain, and this makes for reduced efficiency of your brain.

Having sugary drinks on an empty stomach, for example, can cause a large blood sugar spike, starting the day off with a sugary muffin, or having a midnight snack that is full of sugar will also cause this yo-yo blood sugar effect. This is because when your body is in a fasted state, which means that there is no food that it is digesting currently, the processes that control our blood sugar are resting. When there is a large influx of sugar then, the body's blood sugar-regulating processes were not already in the works, and they will have to not only start up but work even harder than normal because the food that has just entered the body is high in refined sugar. The body makes these levels drop to deal with this and thus begins the yo-yo effect of blood sugar.

This yo-yo of blood sugar levels can lead to rapid changes in mood and rapid rises and falls in energy levels. If you have ever felt a "sugar high," and then shortly after felt like your energy levels fell drastically or you "crashed," this is the effect that you were feeling.

This effect is related to inflammation, and this is a common effect in today's societies because of the mass amounts of sugar that is consumed in our diets.

- **Diet Choice**

There are many foods that are commonly eaten today, which are known to cause inflammation in the body. We will look at this later on in this book so that you can get a better idea of what kinds of foods these are. A poor diet has been shown to lead to a consistent level of low-grade inflammation in the human body. Over time, this inflammation can lead to inflammatory diseases such as obesity, stroke, heart disease, and so on.

- **Allergens**

The chronic inflammation that characterizes these conditions can be caused by environmental factors such as pollution in the air or chronic mold exposure.

- **Long-Term Chemical Exposure**

If you live or work somewhere where you are being exposed to chronic, low-grade chemicals, this could lead to an allergic reaction in the form of chronic inflammation. This can be difficult to notice, as it could leave you simply feeling "off" without knowing exactly why. Be aware of this one so that you can look out for it in your life and in the lives of those you care about.

- **Autoimmune Diseases**

Autoimmune diseases involve the immune system attacking the body, which leads to chronic inflammation, and along with it, a variety of symptoms.

- **Genetics**

Genetics could play a role in a person's chronic inflammation since it can impact things like your risk for obesity or your propensity for alcohol use.

The Science of How Inflammation Is Caused?

Inflammation is a response intended to protect us from whatever signaled the inflammation to occur. It does this by increasing the number of inflammatory cells in the area where the irritant or pathogen is located. The inflammatory cells are there to remove the irritant, promote new cell growth to replace cells that were damaged by the irritant, and then to promote overall repair of the area.

Inflammation and Autophagy

In this section, we are going to look at the science of inflammation and how it is caused by looking at something called *Autophagy*. Autophagy is a process that occurs within the human body. This process has been going on in the cells of the human body since the beginning of us. However, It is only recently that scientists have begun to actually understand this process and how it can help us to learn more about inflammation.

Autophagy, as a word, can be broken up into two individual parts. Each of these parts on its own is a separate Greek word. The word auto means *self* and the word phagy means *the practice of eating*. Putting these together gives you *the practice of self-eating,* which is essentially what autophagy is. Autophagy is the body's way of cleaning itself out. The process involves small "hunter" particles that go around your body looking for cells or cell components that are old and damaged. The hunter particles then take these cell components apart, getting rid of the damaged parts and saving the useful parts to make new cells later. These hunter cells can also use useful leftover parts to create energy for the body.

Autophagy plays a large role in inflammation. Inflammation involves cells in this body being sent to specific locations where they are needed. Once there, they will help to clear the area of damage or intruders, or to help promote healing. Autophagy has a direct impact on these inflammatory cells in the body. Autophagy has the ability to keep inflammatory cells alive by breaking down the old and damaged parts within these inflammatory cells, thus keeping the cells healthy and in good working order for longer. This results in longer inflammation at that specific site within the body.

It does this in the same way that it keeps any of our other cells working and alive. These inflammatory cells are necessary to keep the human body healthy by reaching the site of damage or disease and clearing it out.

The inflammatory cells have many jobs to do in our bodies, so it is important that they stay healthy and are working properly. Autophagy ensures that they can do so, and thus it has a big impact on the overall health of any human being.

One other function that autophagy serves in the human body is helping cells to carry out their death when it is time for them to die. There are times when cells are programmed to die, because of a number of different factors such as age, or the fact that they are not needed anymore. Autophagy will help to kill off cells so that they can be replaced with new, healthy cells. Sometimes these cells need assistance to carry out their programmed death when it is time, and autophagy can help them to do this by breaking them down, as well as helping to clean up any leftover debris around the area after their death. The human body is all about life and death, and these processes are continually going on without our knowledge to keep us healthy and in good form.

Autophagy plays an important role in reducing inflammation as well as causing it, especially in the brain. Since autophagy has the ability to both keep cells alive and to cause their death, it can control the presence of inflammatory cells and control their exit when the irritant has been removed. This is why it is so beneficial at keeping us healthy, as it is needed in order to help you heal and then get you back to normal once you have healed. In the next section, we are going to look at what can happen when this inflammation does not stop. This can happen when those inflammatory cells stay around for much longer than they are needed and do not exit when it is their time.

Chronic Inflammation Versus Acute Inflammation

There are two different types of inflammation. The first one we will discuss is the one you are likely most familiar with, acute inflammation. Then, we will discuss chronic inflammation and how these two types of inflammation differ.

- **Acute Inflammation**

Acute inflammation has a rapid onset but usually only lasts until the bacteria or the injury is gone. Examples of this include a cut or scrape, tonsillitis, sinusitis, and bronchitis. The inflammatory response occurs at the first sign of infection or virus in the body, and these inflammatory cells are no longer present after they have successfully gotten rid of the problem in that area of the body. This is because they are broken down or ushered out when they are no longer needed.

Think about when you have a scrape on your knee from falling. At first, it is red and painful and likely swollen. Over time, as your scrape heals, this redness, pain, and swelling will greatly decrease, and eventually, you will no longer see any sign of a scrape or inflammation at all.

The above example is what it looks like when inflammation is carried out successfully and does its job, before leaving at returning your body back to its normal state.

- **Chronic Inflammation**

The other type of inflammation is chronic inflammation. Chronic inflammation occurs over a long period of time, from months to years, and has a slower onset than acute inflammation. Acute inflammation can become chronic inflammation if the infection or the injury is not resolved as a result of the initial inflammatory immune response. Chronic inflammation can also occur because of consistent exposure over a long period of time to a small amount of an irritant such as allergens or chemicals of some sort. This is because your body will not be able to recognize the absence of the irritant that would signal for the inflammatory cells to leave the area since the person is being exposed over and over again to the same irritant. When inflammation becomes chronic, we begin to see diseases develop.

Inflammation and the Immune System

The way that autophagy assists the immune system is similar to the way in which it helps a damaged or dying cell to complete its cell death or the way in which it helps the human body by keeping cells healthy on a daily basis.

When there is a disease present, the immune system begins to act in the area where the disease or damage is present. Think about when you have had an injury that nearly became infected- it was your immune system that got rid of the infection so that the wound could properly heal without becoming worse.

When the immune system is activated in that area, the disease will be taken up in a pocket created by the cell, and it will be taken to a specific location in the cell where it will be broken down and destroyed.

By this process, the cell is able to get rid of the diseases that have infected it, using the body's immune response. The immune response can be very large or very small, depending on the level of infection, or the amount of disease in the body.

On the other hand, inflammation and the immune system can actually begin to work together against a person's body by way of something called an *Autoimmune Disease*. Autoimmune diseases are diseases caused by the immune system and the body's inflammation response, which together begin attacking the body itself and the tissues of the body. It does this because it begins to mistake them for damaged or diseased tissues, and as a result, it begins to break down and attack cells and tissues that are healthy.

The body confuses unhealthy cells and healthy cells. This can lead to a variety of diseases depending on where in the body this occurs.

Autophagy's role in autoimmune diseases is that it keeps the immune cells healthy and strong. Still, when these cells are not needed, autophagy can end up working against the body as the inflammation becomes painful.

Inflammation and Longevity

Inflammation is essential for the longevity of a person. Autophagy has been shown to have positive effects on aging, and this is why it plays such a large role in longevity. The reason for this is twofold.

The first reason is that the cells that it impacts the most are often damaged or injured. By way of inflammation and autophagy, the disease or infection that is attempting to infect the body is unable to spread, allowing the person to continue living a relatively healthy life. This type of disease and infection control and elimination increases the longevity of the person.

The second reason is that inflammation is essential in maintaining the health of specific tissues and organs within your body, which keeps them working effectively and functioning at their best. This, in turn, is another factor that influences lifespan for the better. If the organs and tissues within a person's body are healthy, the person as a whole will be healthy and will keep living.

In these two ways, inflammation plays a significant role in the longevity and lifespan of a person and their cells.

On the other hand, though, if a person becomes plagued with a disease that involves a malfunction related to inflammation, their lifespan could be reduced greatly.

Inflammation and Quality of Life

While at first inflammation may seem like it has nothing to do with a person's quality of life, it has many indirect effects on the potential for quality of life of any person. Everyone will experience inflammation at some point in their lives. Still, when it begins to become overactive or malfunction, this is when it can cause a lot of problems and impact a person's quality of life in a negative way.

As you have seen in this chapter, and as you will see in the next chapter, inflammation has the potential to affect the body in many positive and negative ways. Autophagy can cause diseases, but it can also prevent them. It has the possibility to maintain and improve the health of a person, but it also has the possibility to create and maintain a state of disease within the body- as you will see in more detail in the next chapter.

Everything in the body comes down to what happens at a cellular level, as the human body works in a bottom-up level of impact. Whatever happens at the cellular level will work its way up, eventually affecting everything at the larger levels, before eventually affecting the human body as a whole. A person will only become aware of what is going on at a cellular level in their body, once its effects have worked their way up to the person's consciousness.

Having a disease, especially one that involves inflammation of some part of the body, can cause high levels of pain and discomfort on a daily basis for the person affected. This affects the quality of life as the person living with pain must take this with them in everything they do. It can cause a person to feel stiffness and high levels of pain in the affected areas, which often prevents them from being able to enjoy activities that they once participated in. When it comes to quality of life, inflammation has been shown to negatively impact mental health as well. The increase of levels of inflammation on a chronic basis within a person's body has been shown to increase instances of depression and food-related disorders such as binge eating.

Remember in chapter one, how we discussed stress and the impacts it has on inflammation within the body? Stress has also been shown to effects people's lives negatively if they already suffer from some type of digestive disorder such as inflammatory bowel disease (IBD) or irritable bowel syndrome (IBS). These two disorders share traits such as constipation, diarrhea, bloating, and stomach pain, which, when experienced over time, will lead to negative consequences for a person's mental health and quality of life.

On the other hand, inflammation can affect the quality of life of a person in a positive way by maintaining their health and eliminating disease. Inflammation in the short term helps to get rid of diseases, bacterial infections, and any sort of injury. By effectively eliminating disease and injury in a timely manner, the person's quality of life is greatly increased as their health is improved.

The effects that inflammation has can be seen as two opposite sides of a coin. For this reason, throughout the rest of this book, we are going to look at a variety of ways that you can take this into your own hands, to avoid having to "flip a coin" when it comes to your longevity. We are going to look at how you can improve your body from the inside in order to live a longer, happier life.

CHAPTER 2

HOW TO TELL IF YOU HAVE CHRONIC INFLAMMATION

In this chapter, we are going to look at the most common signs and symptoms of inflammation so that you can begin to examine your own life and your own body in order to see if you may be suffering from chronic inflammation. We will begin by looking at the symptoms, and then we will discuss the consequences that chronic inflammation can have for your body.

The Signs and Symptoms of Inflammation

There are several common signs that inflammation can be identified in the human body. In this section, we will look at those signs and symptoms.

On the outside of the body, inflammation can be identified by five symptoms. These five symptoms of inflammation are the following:

- Redness
- Swelling
- Heat to the touch
- Pain
- Impaired function of the area

These symptoms are most common among acute instances of inflammation. As you know, inflammation such as this can happen when there is an infection, a physical injury, or if there has been any other assault to that area. If you notice these symptoms in a certain area of your body, there is something going on in that spot which is requiring a response from your immune system in the form of inflammation.

Sometimes, inflammation can occur in the digestive tract as well. There are many symptoms that the inflammation of the digestive tract can be identified by, including the following:

- Nausea
- A lack of appetite
- Fever
- Fatigue
- Abnormal stools

This inflammation in the digestive tract could come about quickly and resolve itself quickly, or it could be chronic and come in the form of Irritable Bowel Disease, in which these symptoms would be a sign of chronic inflammation of the bowels. The symptoms listed in this section are most often seen with acute inflammation, such as when there is a cut or an infection. Later in this chapter, we will look at the common symptoms of chronic inflammation.

Below are the most common signs and symptoms of chronic inflammation. Chronic inflammation can be a much more subtle experience, which can make it hard to identify. These symptoms can last for months or even years before people identify them to be related to chronic inflammation, so being aware of them is important for noticing if you may have some kind of chronic inflammation going on in your body. The most common symptoms of chronic inflammation are the following:

- Fatigue
- Abdominal pain
- Fever
- Rash
- Chest pain
- Mouth sores

Inflammation in the long-term or chronic inflammation can become quite problematic for a person's body, not only on the inside but on the outside as well. When a person is suffering from chronic inflammation, they may experience any or all of the following consequences and symptoms.

- Body pains
- Frequent infections
- Depression
- Anxiety
- Other mood disorders
- Insomnia
- Fatigue
- Weight gain
- Constipation
- Acid reflux
- Diarrhea

There are other common symptoms that can vary depending on the specific area of the body that is experiencing chronic inflammation. For example, if a person has Rheumatoid Arthritis, they will experience inflammation of their joints. This inflammation of the joints is accompanied by the following symptoms:

- Pain in the joints
- Swelling
- Fatigue

- Reduced flexibility and range of motion in the joint
- Stiffness
- Loss of functioning of the joint
- Tingling and numbness

Consequences of Chronic Inflammation in the Body

Inflammation is beneficial and necessary for proper healing and maintenance of good health, but when it occurs over a long period of time (such as years), this lasting amount of inflammation can actually create problems in the body.

As I mentioned, autoimmune diseases are diseases caused by the immune system and the inflammation response of the body, beginning to attack itself and the tissues of the body that are healthy. This causes the body to damage and destroys its own tissues and cells that are in regular working order that would not otherwise be involved in an immune attack. These immune attacks involve inflammatory cells being sent to the area of attack in an effort to rid the body of damage or disease when, in fact, there is no damage or disease to get rid of. As a result of this, there are several consequences for a person's body. These consequences are characterized by specific autoimmune diseases, but for the most part, they all involve pain, swelling, and overall discomfort. We will look at these diseases in more detail in chapter three of this book.

Over time, chronic inflammation will have long-term negative effects on the body. This is because inflammation that is present over a long period of time can actually begin to cause damage to certain parts of the body. For example, chronic inflammation can lead to the damage of healthy tissues and, eventually, the death of these tissues. It can also lead to the damage of healthy organs in the body. These healthy organs can then begin to reduce in function, and this can, in turn, lead to other issues related to impaired organ function. Chronic inflammation can also lead to scarring within the body, and scar tissue being present can cause a number of issues internally. Another known consequence of chronic inflammation is DNA damage, which can then lead to the development of cancer and other degenerative diseases like Alzheimer's and Dementia. Chronic inflammation, in some cases, can even lead to Type 2 diabetes, which is also linked to obesity.

Consequences of Chronic Inflammation in the Brain

An example of chronic inflammation in the brain is the disease called Multiple Sclerosis, or MS. This disease is another example of an autoimmune disorder that results in a chronic immune response and, thus, chronic inflammation. The symptoms of this type of chronic inflammation include the following:

- Balance issues
- Tingling and numbness in the legs, arms or face
- Fatigue
- Vision problems such as blurry vision or vision loss
- Brain fog or cognitive impairment

Another example of chronic inflammation in the brain and the long-term effects it can have include degeneration of the nerves in the brain and damage of the DNA, which can lead to brain-related disorders like dementia.

How Chronic Inflammation Can Affect Your Life

Chronic inflammation can become quite painful. It can cause a person to feel stiffness and high levels of pain in the affected areas. This can lead to a variety of negative impacts on a person's lifestyle. For one, a person can begin to feel self-conscious about their condition. They may experience embarrassment about it, and this can lead to a reduction in social contact. As a result, a person could become isolated, which can then lead to a sedentary lifestyle, which can then increase inflammation. This functions in a cycle that can leave a person feeling dejected and depressed over time.

This is only one example of the way that chronic inflammation can affect a person's life and one piece of evidence as to why this is a widespread problem in the world that must be addressed. By reading this book, you are already on your way to doing so, and throughout the rest of these chapters, I will teach you how.

CHAPTER 3

INFLAMMATORY DISEASES

"Inflammatory Disease" is an umbrella term for a variety of diseases that involve inflammation in some parts of the body, usually experienced over a long period of time. We are going to look at several examples of these diseases in this chapter and how they are caused.

Inflammatory Disease Examples

We are going to begin this chapter by looking at several of the most common diseases that are related to chronic inflammation. These diseases are called inflammatory diseases.

- Chronic Allergies or Hay Fever

Allergies to something like a cat when you visit

someone's house can come about quickly when in the presence of the cat and be gone after a few days once the irritant is removed. Sometimes, however, the inflammation caused by allergies can become chronic and can lead to a condition like hay fever.

- Inflammatory Bowel Disease (IBD)

Inflammatory Bowel Disease is another disease caused by chronic inflammation, and within the term Inflammatory bowel disease (IBD), there are a number of more specific conditions, such as Crohn's Disease.

- Celiac Disease

Celiac disease is a sensitivity in the intestines to gluten. This sensitivity to gluten leads to chronic inflammation of the digestive tract.

- Autoimmune Diseases

There are no known cures for these diseases, and they can only be mediated by symptom-managing treatments. There are a variety of autoimmune diseases that are common in today's society, some of which are listed below.

  - Rheumatoid Arthritis
  - Psoriasis

- Asthma

Asthma is characterized by inflammation of the pathways within the lungs in which air travels when it is breathed in. The inflammation of these tubes leads to people having trouble breathing, as the tubes are constricted.

- Chronic Obstructive Pulmonary Disease or COPD

COPD is another example of a disease that involves a constriction of the lung pathways. COPD can also be considered to be chronic bronchitis, which involves mucus in the lungs. Many people require oxygen 24/7 when they suffer from COPD, and it is often caused by smoking over a long-term basis.

Inflammatory Diseases in the Brain

- Dementia and Alzheimer's Disease

Dementia is a blanket term for a combination of symptoms of cognitive decline, such as forgetfulness and disorientation. Alzheimer's disease is one common example of dementia.

- Stroke

Strokes have been known to be a result of inflammation in many cases, particularly within the United States. This could be associated with a poor diet, for example. In many cases, blood flow to the brain is reduced because of clogged arteries. These clogged arteries do not allow enough blood to flow to the brain, which results in some of the brain cells dying. The death of brain cells signals an immune response in the brain, which leads to inflammation around the site. This inflammation actually works against a person, as the inflammation can further inhibit proper blood flow to the brain, resulting in a stroke.

- Multiple Sclerosis (MS)

An example of chronic inflammation in the brain is the disease called Multiple Sclerosis, or MS. This disease is another example of an autoimmune disorder that results in a chronic immune response and, thus, chronic inflammation.

This autoimmune disease involves an immune attack on the nerve cells in the brain and the spinal cord, resulting in damage to the eyes, the muscles and the overall functioning of the body and a person's ability to control their body systems. This disease can become debilitating for a person suffering from it.

How These Inflammatory Diseases Are Caused

In this section, we will look at the diseases which we discussed above, but in this section, we are going to look at the science of how they are caused and how they can come about in the body.

- How Hay Fever is Caused

This is when the nasal pathways become inflamed in an effort to protect the person from inhaling any more of the irritant (like pollen or grass); however, after a few weeks, this inflammation can become quite irritating to the person experiencing it. They will experience things like a stuffed nose, which can make it difficult for the person to go about their regular lives. At this point, inflammation that is supposed to help the person becomes more of a burden.

- How Asthma is Caused

Asthma is a disease that is caused by inflammation of the tubes that connect and move air to and from the lungs, as well as the tubes within the lungs. Because these airways are inflamed, they are extra sensitive to everything that the lungs inhale, especially irritants of any sort. When an irritant is inhaled, the already inflamed airways become even more swollen, which makes it very difficult for the person to breathe. Asthma and allergies are closely linked and can act in similar ways or in tandem in the body.

- How Inflammatory Bowel Disease is Caused

All of the more specific diseases under this umbrella term are characterized by the inflammation of the digestive tract. IBD is caused by an abnormal response in the gut to certain foods, or bacteria and viruses, leading to chronic inflammation.

- How Rheumatoid Arthritis is Caused

Rheumatoid arthritis is an example of chronic inflammation that becomes quite painful for the person experiencing it. This is due to the fact that the person is experiencing a self-attack from their immune system and chronic inflammation as a result of this. The inflammation that this causes affects a person's joints. Chronic inflammation can become quite painful. Rheumatoid arthritis affects the joints of the body, often in the fingers, wrists, and knees. In this disease specifically, the immune system begins to attack the lining around a joint, and this also causes the joint to become inflamed. This inflammation after a long while can also begin to affect the joint's shape and structure as a whole.

- How Psoriasis is Caused

Psoriasis is another autoimmune condition, this time affecting the skin. This autoimmune response causes extra growth of skin, which leads to the dry and scaly appearance of psoriasis. In this condition, the immune system acts as if it is healing a wound on the skin, sending inflammatory cells, and creating many new skin cells. The problem is that there is no wound to heal, so the skin ends up being inflamed, and the overgrowth of skin cells on top of those that were healthy, to begin with, can be itchy and painful for the person. The body is unable to discern whether there is a wound or not, leading to chronic inflammation.

- How Dementia is Caused

One cause of dementia is cell death, which we know by now involves autophagy. This brain cell death happens over a period of time and includes gradual cognitive decline as this happens. The actual causes of dementia, including Alzheimer's, are not well known, but what is known is that this steady decline is linked to abnormal cell death.

As we saw earlier, when a cell is damaged or infected beyond repair, autophagy is supposed to lead the cell to die, in order to preserve the health of the human being and provide it with a new, healthy cell to take its place.

In other cases, the cell death is programmed, and autophagy begins when this programmed cell death is signaled. This is so that new cells can be created to take their place. Sometimes though, as in the case of dementia, cell death occurs similarly to an autoimmune disorder when it is unprogrammed and unwarranted. In this way, inflammatory cells and autophagy are present at a site where it is not needed, leading to negative effects for the human body. When this happens in the brain, the results are quite damaging to the person's mind.

Other Diseases That Involve Inflammation

- Cancer

Cancer is another umbrella term that includes the entire body. There are numerous types of cancers, but they are all based on the same type of dysfunction of the body's cells. Cancer is caused by malfunctions in the growth of cells, either the uncontrolled growth of new cells or the dramatic slowing of the growth of new cells. Sometimes, this rapid increase in cell creation can cause a tumor, but not all cancers involve tumors. As I mentioned earlier in this book, cell death is a normal part of the body's functioning, and autophagy plays a part in this process. Sometimes, this cell death is not properly executed or communicated, and the cells that are meant to die off and be replaced by new ones do not begin the process of cell death. Because of this, there is a large buildup of cells that begin stealing the nutrients and energy from the other cells that were meant to take their place, and the body begins to experience impaired immune function as well as other malfunctions.

Cancer cells are able to manipulate autophagy to make it work for them when they need and not when they don't need. Cancer cells use autophagy to their benefit by using the breakdown and energy generation to make energy for themselves to thrive and survive in a nutrient-poor environment. The environment within tumors is nutrient-poor because of the large irregular number of cells that must use a regular amount of nutrients. Then, the autophagy is taken advantage of by being used to create nutrients from nothing, by breaking down cell components.

- Obesity

While there can be many causes of obesity, one of the more recently discovered and more recently prevalent causes may be related to inflammation and autophagy or, rather, dysfunction of these processes within the body. This is because of the way that the metabolism is affected.

The body's *Metabolism* is an umbrella term that describes the creation of energy for the body to use in order to do things such as a walk or breathe. It creates this energy by breaking down one thing in order to create energy as a result. The process of breaking things down in order to create energy is called the body's metabolism. There are many different ways that the body gets its energy and many different ways that it breaks down materials in order to get this energy, but they all fall under the umbrella of metabolism. In more specific terms, the metabolism is all of the processes in your body that work together to maintain your life.

For example, this happens when you eat food, and it is broken down in your stomach and intestines to create energy for your body to function. This is why we need to eat food in order to stay alive.

This also happens on a smaller scale in each cell of your body using the process of autophagy, as it carries broken or old cell parts to something called *the lysosome* where they are broken down. The breakdown of these cell components is used to create energy for the cell and for your body as a whole.

When a person is running low on energy, a signal is sent within the cells of the body, which tells them to begin breaking down old cell parts for energy, thus creating energy for that cell and for the body.

When cells are experiencing a lack of nutrition and autophagy is triggered, there is also a release of hormones by the body that accompanies this, in an effort to use the energy that it has created in the most efficient way possible. The hormones that are released make the body's fat storage centers more easily broken down and more accessible to the body's metabolism so that they can be used as a source of energy. Because of this, the body's rate of metabolism increases during these times of cellular starvation.

The problem that can occur, which can lead to obesity, is that autophagy becomes improperly regulated within the cells. This means that the cell could have trouble getting autophagy started, or it could have trouble signaling the release of hormones that would make the body break down its fat stores for energy. If this is the case, it can lead to a variety of metabolic disorders, obesity being one of them. This is most often caused by problems related to autophagy's functioning in fat tissues, especially, which then leads to problems in the breakdown of fat tissues and an inability to lose weight in the form of fat. This can then lead a person to continue putting on weight and being unable to lose it.

Fat tissues in the body are also known to include a variety of immune cells. These immune cells are in constant conversation with fat cells, and together they are able to regulate immune responses. Sometimes, when there are too many fat cells, they experience a reduction in proper blood flow, and this can lead them to malfunction. This malfunction results in the overactivity of immune cells, which leads to inflammation. In this way, obesity and inflammation are closely related. In order to deal with the inflammation, it is necessary to deal with obesity, which is why we are going to spend ample time in this book looking at how you can change your diet for the better.

- Heart Disease

Heart disease is an umbrella term for diseases that involve the heart itself or the blood vessels, veins, and arteries that are connected to it. Under this term, the diseases included are coronary heart disease, arrhythmia, heart failure, stroke, and heart attack. These diseases are related to inflammation as they involve inflammation of the structures around the heart, which can lead to blood clots, blockages, or abnormal functioning of the heart and the blood vessels.

- Type 2 Diabetes

Diabetes involves a problem with the body's ability to use insulin. Insulin allows the body to use the sugar that is taken into the body for things such as energy production. When there is a problem with this, it leads to inflammation. In turn, this inflammation makes it harder for the body to respond to insulin, causing more inflammation. This leads to a vicious cycle of insulin resistance and inflammation, and it can make type 2 diabetes worse over time.

The Importance of Preventing Inflammation

As you may have noticed, many of these diseases go hand in hand with one another. If you have one of these diseases, it can lead to a higher risk of developing one or more additional diseases related to inflammation. For example, if you have a disease such as obesity, it can lead you to develop type 2 diabetes. These two diseases can also increase your risk of developing some type of heart disease. All three of these diseases involve chronic inflammation, both as their cause and their symptoms. This leads to increased inflammation.

For this reason, it is important to get ahead of chronic inflammation before it develops. This can reduce your risk of developing not only one single disease, but a whole host of inflammatory diseases.

The Science of How Inflammation Can Be Prevented

Inflammation can be prevented in numerous ways, but the most basic way to reduce inflammation is to provide your body with an environment that is clean, healthy, and free of chemicals and additives. These can be found in food, in cigarettes, in alcohol, and so on. Your body has a difficult time discerning whether you are giving it these things on purpose or whether it is experiencing a sort of "attack of poison," so it responds in the same way regardless. This response involves inflammation. For this reason, you must keep your body healthy and clear of chemical additives such as refined sugar, trans fats, and other ingredients commonly found in food that we eat in today's world.

In the next chapter, we are going to look at the anti-inflammatory diet, which is the key to providing your body with this ideal environment for health and inflammation reduction. Before moving on, though, we are going to discuss two other ways that inflammation can be prevented.

There are two additional ways to prevent or decrease inflammation. These two ways are through regular exercise and through adequate restful sleep.

- Exercise

Exercising regularly has been shown to reduce inflammation, as it actually reduces the number of something called *inflammatory markers* in your body. What this means is that there is less instance of chronic and general inflammation in people who follow a regular and consistent exercise regime.

Further, aerobic exercise has been shown through studies to increase autophagy in the cells of the muscles, the heart, the brain, lungs, and the liver.

When we do aerobic exercise, the heart and lungs work with the muscles to move the body in a specific way (like running or biking). Over time, the heart, lungs, and brain will learn to function together more efficiently, which is why exercises get easier the more you do them. Autophagy is upregulated in these specific tissues (heart, lungs, muscles) after aerobic exercise because these are the specific tissues most positively affected by aerobic exercise. What this means is that since autophagy is increased in these tissues after aerobic exercise, these specific tissues will experience a reduction in inflammation, since autophagy helps to clear out inflammatory cells, as you learned earlier on in this book.

- Restful sleep

Sleep is very important for autophagy as well, just like exercise is. If you have ever gone a few days without a proper, restful sleep, you know that you begin to feel a decline in your mental abilities rather quickly. This could be because of your brain's decreased autophagy functioning.

The number of hours that you are in bed does not matter if the sleep is not good quality. Quality sleep for the right number of hours is what is needed to maintain good brain function and keep your brain's autophagy going. What this does is keep the cells of your brain healthy and clear of any debris, and this includes clearing out the inflammatory cells that are not serving any purpose any longer.

When it is dark outside, there are processes that happen within your brain that tell the body it is time to wind down for sleep. It is at this time that the hormone Melatonin is released in your brain. You may have heard of melatonin before or seen it in pill-form at the drug store. The release of Melatonin is what makes you feel tired in the evening around your "bedtime." Melatonin helps you to fall asleep and to stay deeply asleep throughout the night. The release of Melatonin is associated with autophagy within the brain, and this is why it is important to maintain a regular, consistent sleep-wake cycle.

If your sleep-wake cycle becomes mixed up by something like shift work or inconsistent sleeping hours, it will make it difficult for the brain to produce and release adequate levels of Melatonin, and they may not be released at the times that you need them. This is why some people choose to take Melatonin as a supplement in order to get their sleep-wake cycle back on track by helping their brain out a little bit. It is important not to take too much melatonin in pill-form, however, as sometimes your brain could begin to rely on its supplementation, and this could disturb the natural production of it in the brain. By helping your body to make adequate melatonin at the right times, you will give yourself the opportunity to have a good, restful sleep, and with this comes the increase of autophagy in the brain and, thus, a reduction in inflammation.

CHAPTER 4

THE ANTI-INFLAMMATORY DIET

In this chapter, we are going to begin talking about The Anti-Inflammatory Diet. This diet has the ability to help you in a number of ways, including improving your health, reducing your risk of disease, and increasing your overall quality of life. Throughout this chapter, we are going to look at the reasons for this and how this diet can give you all of these benefits and more.

What Is the Anti-Inflammatory Diet?

There are some foods which are known to increase inflammation in the body, and others that are known to decrease it. The basic premise of the anti-inflammatory diet involves sticking to those foods that are known to decrease inflammation and stay away from those that are known to increase it.

This diet came about because of the recent scientific research findings that state that the vast majority of diseases that lead to death in today's society are related to inflammation. That is to say; they are some type of disease included under the umbrella term Inflammatory Disease. Because this has become such a problem in the United States, especially over the past decade, scientists and nutritionists are interested in finding out how this can be improved and resolved so that we lose fewer lives to preventable diseases related to inflammation.

Findings have shown that by following a diet rich in anti-inflammatory foods, a person is able to reduce chronic inflammation, thereby reducing their risk of and symptoms of inflammatory diseases.

What Are the Benefits of an Anti-Inflammatory Diet?

There are numerous benefits to following an anti-inflammatory diet, whether you are already suffering from an inflammatory disease or not. Below, I have outlined several of these benefits.

- Prevent diseases

As I mentioned, the anti-inflammatory diet is beneficial for preventing a number of diseases. We will look at these diseases later on in this chapter.

- Prevent additional diseases

Inflammatory disease usually come about in groups. This is because the causes of one usually lead to another, which leads to another, and so on. For this reason, it is important to prevent any further inflammatory diseases from developing, especially if you already suffer from one or more of them. The anti-inflammatory diet will help you to do so.

- Deal with symptoms of the disease

If you are dealing with the symptoms of an inflammatory condition such as arthritis or obesity, you will be able to find some level of relief from the associated symptoms such as pain or swelling by following an anti-inflammatory diet for a sustained period of time.

- Lose weight

Losing weight is not an easy task, but by following this diet, you will be able to set yourself up for success in terms of weight loss by reducing the amount of calorie-dense, nutrient-limited foods that you ingest. You will find examples of this in the following chapter.

- Improve overall health

By improving your diet, you not only reduce your risk of disease, but you also improve your life and your level of health overall. The longer you stick to this diet, the more numerous the benefits will be.

Who Should Follow the Anti-Inflammatory Diet?

The anti-inflammatory diet is for anyone who wants to begin changing their life and their body for the better! There is no one specific group of people that this diet is designed to help, as this will help anyone and everyone. Instead of being a fad diet, this way of eating will simply take you back to a more traditional form of eating- one that includes healthy, whole foods. These types of foods are beneficial for anyone and everyone, especially those who are predisposed to certain health conditions, or those who are already suffering from a disease related to inflammation such as heart disease or obesity. This is especially true for those who follow certain lifestyle habits such as smoking or drinking alcohol excessively.

These diseases do not discriminate based on genetics. They will reach anyone who is living a lifestyle that is not conducive to health and physical wellness. For this reason, anyone and everyone should begin to see that the way we eat in this world today is not beneficial for our bodies and that something must be done about it. That something is the anti-inflammatory diet.

What Diseases Does This Diet Help?

- Crohn's Disease

One example of an IBD is Crohn's Disease, where any part of the digestive tract can be the site of inflammation. The food that a person puts in their body is very important when they have IBD, as the food will have to go through the digestive tract, and thus the inflamed areas will be involved every time the person ingests food. By improving your diet and including only anti-inflammatory foods, you will be able to reduce your risk of this disease or improve the symptoms of it if you are suffering from it already.

- Cancer

Remember earlier in this book, how we discussed something called autophagy? Here we will revisit it again, as it can be impacted by a person's diet. Increasing autophagy within the body can actually reduce a person's risk of cancer. This can be done by eating certain foods that are known to increase autophagy in the body. This is because of the way that it is able to clear the body of damaged cells. When damaged cells multiply and divide, this can cause a buildup that can become dangerous and eventually cancerous. If autophagy is functioning properly, it should be able to break down these cells before they can build up, and in this way, autophagy keeps a person healthy and cancer-free.

It is for this reason that many people are choosing to take this into their own hands and trigger autophagy within their cells by following an anti-inflammatory diet, as this is one of the many things that this diet can do for you.

In addition to triggering Autophagy in your body, there are many ways that you can help to reduce your risk of Cancer through dietary means by following the anti-inflammatory diet. There are many bioactive compounds in food that can reduce your risk of developing cancer. These compounds are things like the following;

- Antioxidants- get rid of harmful by-products produced by damaged cells, clearing out the harmful clutter and debris in the body.
- 6-Shogaol- Found in ginger and is known to

be anti-inflammatory, pain-relieving, and nausea-reducing.

* Phytochemicals- Chemicals found in plants that act positively in the body to produce health benefits. Found in vegetables.

These cancer-fighting compounds can be found in plant-based whole foods like Garlic, Ginger, Carrots, Broccoli, tomatoes, dark chocolate, green tea, and so on. This is why eating, according to an anti-inflammatory diet, is so beneficial for reducing your risk of developing cancer.

* Alzheimer's

There are some foods that you should include in your diet if you want to reduce your risk of developing Alzheimer's disease. These foods contain brain cell-preserving compounds which help to keep the brain cells healthy and reduce the chances of dementia. Some of these compounds and foods that they can be found in are listed below;

* Omega 3 Fatty Acids- Improve cognitive function and reduce inflammation in the brain
* Brussels sprouts, cabbage, Kale – Sulforaphane which is a dementia-slowing phytochemical that acts by protecting the brain cells
* Coffee and the Coffee Cherry- caffeine and

antioxidants that are beneficial for brain health
- Green Tea- helps with memory and learning
- Coconut oil- increases Ketosis in the brain leading to better brain health
- Reishi Mushrooms- improve immune function, brain function
- Turmeric- protects the brain cells from damage
- Extra Virgin olive Oil- slows the progression of Alzheimer's

Notice that all of the foods listed above are contained within the parameters of an anti-inflammatory diet. These foods can and should all be ingested regularly when following the anti-inflammatory diet in order to prevent Dementia and Alzheimer's.

Scientific Research About the Anti-Inflammatory Diet

The anti-inflammatory diet works with the latest research in human health to develop an easy to follow diet that is full of delicious food options for you. This diet works in combination with the natural functioning of the human body, which works by way of a simple mathematic equation. The foods that you eat when you are following the anti-inflammatory diet will have a profound impact on your success in terms of weight loss and disease prevention.

This is because if you turn to calorie-dense and

nutrient-sparse foods in high quantities (such as foods high in refined sugar or trans fats), you may not end up with a calorie deficit at the end of the day or at the end of the week.

What this means is that if you are following the anti-inflammatory diet as a method of weight loss or in order to prevent obesity, you will need to ensure that you understand the following scientific concept. The basic equation to represent this concept will be;

The number of calories that you ingest – (minus) The number of calories you use to survive (for example, walking, eating, breathing) - (minus) The extra calories burned from exercise = (equals)

The number that results from this equation (in the equals position) will either be a positive number or a negative number.

- If the number is positive, this means that you ingested more calories than you burned. If the number is positive, you can envision it like having more energy than you were able to use. When this occurs, the extra energy is stored as fat in the body.
- If the number is negative, this means that you burned more calories than you ingested. If the number is negative, you used more energy than you had, and this translates to weight loss.

This is because once the readily available energy in your body is all used up, the body's fat storage will begin to be used for additional energy, resulting in a loss of weight in the form of fat.

- If the number is zero, this means that calories ingested and calories burned are equal to one another. If the number is zero, this indicates "breaking even" in terms of your energy.

This equation explains how falling off of the diet for one meal or two each day could lead to a maintenance of the same weight or even an increase in weight in some cases. If you are using the anti-inflammatory diet as a means of improved health, then this will be a little different for you, but in general, in order to improve your health by way of this diet, you want to achieve either a zero value or a caloric deficit as a result of this equation.

How This Diet Will Improve a Person's Life

If you are someone who experiences chronic inflammation, you likely know how difficult it is to live with it day in and day out. If you are not this type of person, maybe you know someone who is.

If you think back on my example from earlier about how a person living with chronic inflammation may feel self-conscious and end up feeling depressed and lonely after some time, we are going to revisit that example here.

Think about this person once again and think about how their life would change if they began following an anti-inflammatory diet. They would not only begin to feel better physically, in terms of their inflamed areas becoming less painful or less swollen, but they would also begin to feel better mentally and emotionally, as they would then begin to feel more confident in themselves, they would begin to socialize more, and overall they would be able to begin living a full life once again. This is the potential of the anti-inflammatory diet.

CHAPTER 5

ANTI-INFLAMMATORY FOODS AND FOODS TO AVOID

Now that you are aware of what exactly the anti-inflammatory diet is, we are going to look at some more specific examples of foods that you can eat and foods that you should avoid. The foods in each of these two categories have been researched and found to either reduce inflammation in the body or increase it, which is why these recommendations are so important for you if you are looking to improve your health by way of inflammation reduction.

Foods to Avoid on the Anti-Inflammatory Diet

We will begin this chapter by looking at the foods that you should avoid on an anti-inflammatory diet, as they have been shown to increase inflammation or lead to a worsening of autoimmune disorders and diseases involving chronic inflammation.

Below are some of the worst culprits when it comes to foods that increase or exacerbate inflammation.

- Sugar
- Alcohol
- Trans Fats
- Processed Meats
- Refined Carbohydrates

At this point in the chapter, we are going to look at the general term that all of the ingredients in the list above fall into. This general term is *Industrial Foods*. These are the foods that are sold and marketed to us that are not considered *whole foods*.

Whole foods are things like fruits, vegetables, lean meats, and things like this that are not created in a factory. These whole foods are healthy and nutritious, whereas industrial foods are the exact opposite of this.

Industrial foods are foods that are processed and made commercially, such as in a factory or some other process of mass-production. These foods include convenience-made foods like pre-packaged foods, snack foods, or foods that are sold to us in fast-food restaurants. These foods are quick consumption foods that are made to be easily prepared or consumed immediately. We will look at the common ingredients in these foods and the reasons why they taste so great to humans. We will look at what they do to our bodies and why they are not the best option for us. Industrial food production is all about convenience, speed, and ease of production, sale, and consumption. These foods are not made with the people who will consume them in mind. They are made with the dollar in mind and are marketed towards us as if they are a good option to save time and still eat all of our meals. We will now look at the most common ingredients you can find in industrially produced foods and what these ingredients actually are. Many times, we may see ingredients on the packages of foods we eat, but we aren't really sure exactly what they are, just that they taste good. In this section, we will go deeper into them.

Food Coloring

Many different food colorings are used in processed foods to give them the visual appeal that will make them look appetizing and make people buy them. The problem here is that these dyes are chemicals that we do not need to be consuming and have been known to cause children to become hyperactive. These dyes are included in mass-produced foods because without them; we would see that most of these processed foods actually look quite unappealing and of sort of greyish-brown color after all of the processing, additions of chemicals and before they have been colored. For example, much of the time when we see a package of "brown bread" we think that this means it is healthier for us. This is not necessarily true though, as sometimes the bread that is brown is actually just white bread or bread with processed flour and many additives that has been colored brown so that we as consumers think it is healthier for us.

MSG

MSG stands for Monosodium Glutamate, which sounds way too science for many of our brains to even pronounce, let alone know what it is or what it does. MSG is added to foods to give it a delicious flavor. It is essentially a very concentrated form of salt. What this does in foods such as fast-food, packaged convenience foods, and buffet-style food is that it gives it that wonderfully salty and fatty flavor that makes us love these foods so much. Companies put this in food because it comes at an extremely low cost, and the flavor it brings covers up the not-so-great flavor of all of the other cheap ingredients that are used to make the food.

MSG has been known to block our natural appetite suppressant chemicals that normally are released when we have had enough to eat. Therefore, when we are eating foods like this, we do not recognize when we are satiated, and we continue to eat it because it tastes so great.

Fat, Salt and Sugar

Now for the trifecta- fat, salt, and sugar are often seen as a triad in the most processed foods. Even if you think a food is very salty, like a fast-food French fry, there are most definitely heaps of sugar added into it as well. While these three being found together make for a great taste for our taste buds, they are not so great for the body. When finding them all together in a single food item, this is what makes your body crave the food over and over again. Fat, salt, and sugar can be found combined as High-Fructose Corn Syrup, as we talked about previously, or as oils that have been hydrogenated or processed heavily. These two ingredients are cheap and flavorful, so they are added to just about everything we buy in fast-food restaurants or heavily processed foods. If you go to a regular sit-down restaurant, they may not be using only industrially-processed foods, but they will be sure to use a large amount of sugar, fat, and salt together in a single dish which is what will make the food taste great and will keep you coming back again and again.

High Fructose Corn Syrup

High fructose corn syrup is surely an ingredient you have heard of before or at least one that you have seen on the packaging of your favorite snacks or quick foods. While this is actually derived from real corn, after it is finished being processed, there is nothing corn-like about it. High fructose corn syrup is essentially the same thing as refined sugar when all is said and done. It is used as a sweetener in foods like soda, cereal, and other sweet and quick foods. The reason why this ingredient is seen so often is that it is much cheaper than using sugar and is much easier to work with.

Preservatives

There are so many preservatives in our foods today and so many different names for them that only the most advanced scientists could pronounce. Preservatives are added to foods in order to keep them fresh for longer or to increase their shelf life. If you have ever seen videos or articles about heavily processed foods that are laughing about how twenty years from now, they will still look exactly the same, and will not have become moldy or decayed at all, this is because of the preservatives added to it. The longer things will last, the more preservatives they have added into them. If you buy fruit or vegetables regularly, you will know that after about a week or so in the fridge, they start to become moldy and decay. This is what a regular whole food would do, but an industrially processed food would not.

Casein

The next ingredient we will look at is called Casein. This is a heavily processed ingredient that is derived from milk- this is where it is naturally found, it is processed a few times over and eventually creates milk solids that are concentrated. This is then added into things like cheese, French fries, milkshakes, and other fast and convenient packaged or fast-food joint foods that contain dairy or dairy products like pastries and dressings. Casein actually is addictive in itself, and this makes the food it is added to quite addictive for us.

Why Are These Foods Addictive?

Now that we have gone through the ingredients that you will see most commonly in industrially produced foods. We will look at their addictive nature and the chemicals and processes in the body that actually make this happen.

To begin, we will return to Casein, the milk-derived ingredient that has highly addictive properties. Casein has been compared to nicotine in its addictive properties. It is often seen in cheese, and this is why there is increasing evidence that people can become, and many are already addicted to cheese. The reason for this is during digestion. When cheese and other foods that contain casein are digested, it is broken down, and one of the compounds that it breaks down into is a compound that is strikingly similar to opioids- the highly addictive substance that is in pain killers.

Combining fat and carbohydrates in foods, such as potato chips, pizza, French fries, etcetera, has been shown to make these foods even more difficult to resist than other foods that do not contain these similar combinations.

High Fructose Corn Syrup has also been shown to be highly addictive. This substance has been shown to be similar to cocaine in its addictive properties.

The reason that these foods are addictive is their chemical structure. A chemical structure is like the organization of the molecules that make something what it is. Everything has its own chemical structure- or its own specific arrangement of molecules, and this is what makes everything different from each other, but some things similar. If two things have very similar chemical structures, they will be similar substances, materials, or objects. So, these addictive chemicals that are found in industrially produced foods are built of a chemical structure that is very similar to the chemical structure of highly addictive drugs like cocaine, heroin, or opioids. Either this or they break down in our digestive system, and then this process creates chemicals that are very similar to the chemical structure of drugs that are highly addictive. So, to understand why these specific chemical structures are addictive, we will have to understand the science of our brains in a little bit more depth. The next section will go deeper into this so that we can understand that we are very susceptible to food addictions, especially of very specific types of foods.

How Are These Foods Like Drugs?

As I mentioned previously, the chemicals that are found in foods like High Fructose Corn Syrup, Casein, Fats, and Salts contain chemical structures that eventually will travel to our brains. When they get there, they find very specific places to rest. These places are built like a puzzle, so these chemicals find their matching puzzle piece in the brain, and they stick to it tightly as their structures fit together perfectly. This is the same with drugs. When we ingest an opioid, like oxycodone, which is a narcotic, this opioid makes its way to the brain and does the same thing. It will look for its matching puzzle piece and link to it tightly. The problem is because the chemicals in food and the chemicals that are highly addictive drugs are very similar; these will find the exact same puzzle pieces as each other. Because of this, they make us feel the same way as each other.

The way that they make us feel is happy, giddy, elated, and like we are having a great time. This feeling is what keeps people who are addicted to these drugs like painkillers or cocaine going back to them for more. This is where the addiction to these drugs comes from. It is more than a conscious decision to continue, but the pursuit of these wonderful feelings that come from a very real chemical reaction in our brain.

Why does this chemical reaction make us feel so good? This is because these drugs act like a reward for the brain and the body. When these chemicals- be they drugs or food additives, find their matching puzzle pieces within the brain, this matching of pieces causes another chemical to be released by the brain. This other chemical that is released is what then makes our brain feel like it has been rewarded. The rewarding feeling makes us feel accomplished, happy, and excited. As humans, receiving the feeling of reward is very strong and very addictive. Every time our brain has this puzzle piece matching, we feel a sense of reward. And whether this comes from a drug or a food additive, our brain can't tell. All our brain knows is that there has been a chemical connection, and it then releases the reward chemical. This is why these addictions are so hard to break. When it comes to drug addictions, people seem to understand that there is something more than the person's willpower involved, and it is something that must be fought hard in order to overcome. The thing that is less understood is that when it comes to food addiction, this is the exact same thing. By explaining this chemical process to you in this chapter, I hope that this helps you to understand why you have a difficult time stopping yourself if you suffer from binge eating, or why it is so hard to say no when you feel like turning to food as a comfort.

Sugar

We will now look more closely at sugar and the ways in which it affects our bodies and our minds. Sugar is actually the worst culprit of all of these food additives. This is because it is so hard to avoid! Sugar is found in everything we eat that we can buy from a restaurant or a store. There are so many forms of sugar and so many names that it is usually disguised in the ingredients list on food packaging. One food may contain 70 percent sugar, but on the label, it may look as if this is not true because the different types of sugar have all been separated in order to trick us into thinking this is not the case. When it comes to avoiding sugar, it takes diligence and a keen eye for detail.

We already discussed one form of sugar, High Fructose Corn Syrup. This type of sugar is cheap and easy to use and is added to virtually everything packaged that we can ingest. This is because it gives even salty foods that tasty flavor balance.

Sugar As a Drug

As we talked about previously in this chapter, the chemicals found in food act in our brains in a very similar way to the way in which highly addictive drugs act. Sugar itself acts in a specific way that makes it so difficult to avoid. Sugar affects what is called the *Limbic System.* The limbic system is a group of structures in the brain that has to do with our emotions and our memory. This includes the regulation of our emotions and forming memories, which contributes to our learning. What this means is that when we eat something very sugary, the chemicals that make up the sugars can affect our emotions. When this happens, it makes us feel emotions like happiness and satisfaction. Then, because eating certain foods makes us feel like this, we form a memory of this, and in turn, we learn that eating these specific foods gives us positive emotions. This makes us keep coming back for more.

So, when we eat something that contains both sugars and Casein, for example, we will get action on our limbic system as well as on our reward system in the brain. Therefore, foods that give us both a feeling of reward and a surge of positive emotion are the most difficult to resist, and the first ones we turn to when we want comfort in the form of food because we know they will make us feel good. And they always do, as these chemical reactions in the brain occur each time. We may not even realize this, as it becomes second nature to us. We may not recognize the positive feelings we get after we eat something that comforts us, but for some reason, we know we keep craving it. If this has ever happened to you, you now know why this is. After learning about these things, pay attention to your cravings and see if this may be the explanation for why you have them. Pay attention also to the times that these cravings occur. Did you just receive some bad news? Was it on a rainy day when you were feeling especially down? Hold onto this information as we will revisit it shortly. Later on, in this book, we will also be discussing several ways to overcome these challenges to break the cycles of emotional eating and overeating.

Examples of Ingredients That Are Anti-Inflammatory

In this section, we are going to look at a number of ingredients that can be found within certain foods that are known to have anti-inflammatory effects in the body. By eating these ingredients, or foods containing them, you will increase the value of this diet for your body.

Bioactive Compounds

Bioactive compounds are compounds found within foods that act in the body in beneficial ways. The bioactive compounds found within berries, such as Acai Berries, Strawberries, and Blueberries are very beneficial for your health. The bioactive compounds in these specific types of berries work in the brain to induce autophagy and reduce inflammation. This leads to the protection of brain cells in this case from *oxidative stress*. Oxidative stress is something that can happen within the brain when there is an imbalance of oxygen, which can cause reduced cognitive functioning. These berries and their induction of autophagy helps to reduce this by keeping the balance of oxygen at a healthy level.

Omega 3 Fatty Acids

These are something that are essential since they

cannot be made in our bodies. Omega-3 Fatty Acids are substances that are necessary to get from your diet as the body cannot make them on its own. These fatty acids are a certain type in a list of other fatty acids, but this type (Omega-3) are the most essential and the most beneficial for our brains and bodies in general. They have numerous effects on the brain, including reducing inflammation (which reduces the risk of Alzheimer's) and maintaining and improving mood and cognitive function, including specifically memory. Omega-3's have these greatly beneficial effects because of the way that they act in the brain, which is what makes them so essential to our diets. Omega-3 Fatty Acids increase the production of new nerve cells in the brain by acting specifically on the nerve stem cells within the brain, causing new and healthy nerve cells to be generated.

Omega-3 fatty acids can be found in fish like salmon, sardines, black cod, and herring. It can also be taken as a pill-form supplement for those who do not eat fish or cannot eat enough of it. It can also be taken in the form of a fish oil supplement like krill oil.

Omega-3's is by far the most important nutrient that you need to ensure you are ingesting because of the numerous benefits that come from it, both in the brain and in the rest of the body. While supplements are often a last step when it comes to trying to include something in your diet, for Omega-3's, the benefits are too great to potentially miss by trying to receive all of it from your diet.

What Kinds of Foods Can You Eat on the Anti-Inflammatory Diet?

- Berries

Berries such as acai berries, strawberries, blackberries, and blueberries are beneficial due to their anti-inflammatory properties, as you have seen above.

- Fruits

Other fruits, in addition to berries are included in the anti-inflammatory diet, as they are naturally occurring in nature and are beneficial for your health in a general sense.

Examples of fruits that you can eat include the following:

- Citrus fruits such as oranges, grapefruits, lemons, and limes
- Melons of a variety of sorts
- Apples
- Bananas
- Berries including strawberries, blueberries, blackberries, raspberries and so on
- Grapes

- Vegetables

Vegetables are a great source of energy and nutrients, and they include a wide range of naturally occurring vivid colors which should all be included in your diet. When choosing vegetables, choose as much variety in terms of color as you can. The great thing about vegetables is that they occupy a lot of space for the number of calories consumed, and they are also packed with nutrients. Adding a number of vegetables that are larger than the size of your fist is going to fill you up without leaving you hungry a short time later and will also be giving you all of the nutrients you need to be a healthy individual.

- Carrots
- Broccoli and cauliflower
- Asparagus
- Kale
- All sorts of peppers including hot peppers, bell peppers
- Tomatoes
- Root vegetables (that are a good source of healthy, complete carbohydrates) such as potatoes, sweet potatoes, all types of squash, and beets.

Fruits and vegetables aren't the only types of foods that you can eat on an anti-inflammatory diet.

There are a variety of other plant-based foods that are included because of their positive effects on your body.

- Legumes

Legumes are a great source of protein as well as fiber, and there are many different types to choose from. These include the following:

- All sorts of beans including black beans, green beans, and kidney beans
- Peas
- Lentils of all colors
- Chickpeas
- Peas
- Protein

The best sources of protein are always going to be the leanest and most natural sources. The less lean forms of meat protein contain lots of animal fat, which is not the good kind of fat we are looking for. Lean meats include turkey, chicken, lean beef and fish

Eggs are a good source of protein as well as dairy sources like milk and cheese. Greek yogurt has a lot of protein and can be bought without added sugar, making it a good choice for a healthy snack. Below, we will look at these lean protein sources in more detail.

Fish is a great way to get healthy fats as well as lean protein when following the anti-inflammatory diet. Certain fish are very low in carbohydrates but high in good fats, making them perfect for your health overall. They also contain minerals and vitamins that will be good for your health. Salmon is a great fish to eat on this diet as it is essentially carbohydrate-free. Many fish also include essential fatty acids that we can only get through our diet. Other fish that are good to eat on the anti-inflammatory diet are:

- Sardines
- Mackerel
- Herring
- Trout
- Albacore Tuna

Meat and Poultry make up a large part of anybody's diet (as long as they are not a vegetarian). Meats and poultry that are fresh and not processed do not include any carbohydrates but contain high levels of protein. Eating lean meats when on the anti-inflammatory diet helps to maintain your strength and will help you to keep your muscle mass, even if you happen to be losing weight. Further, if you have decreased your carbohydrate intake significantly, eating meat will help you to keep your body strong. Grass-fed meats, in particular, are rich in antioxidants and beneficial fats, which is great for combatting inflammation on this diet.

Eggs are another amazing anti-inflammatory food. They have virtually no carbohydrates and contain protein. Eggs help you to feel full for longer and keep blood sugar levels consistent, which is great for overall health and for combatting obesity. The whole egg is good for you, as the yolk is where the nutrients are. The cholesterol found within egg yolks also has been shown to reduce the risk of heart disease, despite what most people think. When on an anti-inflammatory diet, do not be afraid of the yolk of the egg. Further, some eggs are fortified with Omega 3 fatty acids, which are great for reducing inflammation and which is an essential nutrient that your body needs.

Greek Yogurt is a food that is high in protein but small amounts of carbohydrates. **Cottage Cheese** is another similar food that contains high protein and low carbohydrates. They both help you to feel full, from eating small amounts and keep you full for longer because of the protein they contain, which keeps giving you energy for a prolonged period. These can be put together with other foods or eaten alone. This is a great way to have a quick snack without turning to sugary or fatty convenience foods.

- Seeds

Seeds are another great source of nutrients, vitamins, and minerals, and they are very versatile. These include the following:

- Sesame seeds
- Pumpkin seeds
- Sunflower seeds
- Hemp, flax and chia seeds are all especially good for your health
- Nuts

Nuts are a great way to get protein if you are choosing not to eat meat or if you are vegan. They also are packed with nutrients. Some examples are below.

- Almonds
- Brazil Nuts
- Cashews
- Macadamia nuts
- Pistachios
- Pecans
- Healthy Fats

There are some **healthy fats** that are essential components of any person's diet, as the beneficial compounds that they contain cannot be made by our bodies. Thus we rely solely on or diet to get them. These compounds are Omega-3 Fatty Acids, monounsaturated and polyunsaturated fats. Below are some healthy sources of these compounds:

- Avocados
- Healthy, plant-based oils including olive oil and canola oil
- Hemp, chia and flax seeds
- Walnuts

You may be wondering what types of fats you can include in your diet that are not bad fats. Some examples of less desirable fats would include chocolate and fats from oils. The types of fat that you can include in amounts the size of your thumb include avocados, nuts like almonds, coconut oil, and other natural sources like this. The key to knowing which ones are to stick to the least amount of processing possible. The closest to the natural form that you would find in nature, the better.

- Whole Grain Carbohydrates

When it comes to carbohydrates, these should be consumed in the form of **whole grains**, as they are high in fiber, which will help to prevent overeating. Whole grains also include essential minerals- those that we can only get from our diet just like those essential compounds found in healthy fats. These essential minerals are selenium, magnesium, and copper. Sources of these whole grains include the following:

- Quinoa
- Rye, Barley, buckwheat
- Whole grain oats
- Brown rice
- Whole grain bread can be hard to find these days in the grocery store, as many brown breads disguise themselves as whole grain when, in fact, they are not. However, there are whole grain breads if you take the time to look at the ingredients list.

- Plant-based milks

Plant-Based milk is another way to eat healthily while having things that require milk or a milk-like substance. These are great if you are dairy-free or vegan, or if you simply prefer to get your milk from a plant source instead of an animal source. Be sure to check the ingredients to see if there are any added chemicals or sugars and try to choose the most natural. Some examples of these include the following:

- Rice milk
- Hemp milk
- Coconut milk

- Almond milk
- Oat milk
- Soy milk

Remember the term *autophagy* that you learned earlier on in this book? To refresh your memory, autophagy will help to kill off cells so that they can be replaced with new, healthy cells- especially when it comes to inflammatory cells. For this reason, if you are able to encourage your body's autophagy processes, you will be able to reduce chronic inflammation in your body. For this reason, in this section, we are going to look at specific foods that are known to induce autophagy in the human body. This, in turn, will have beneficial effects on inflammation.

- Coffee

It may come as a surprise, but coffee and caffeine, in general, have been shown to induce autophagy, specifically within the brain. It is not only the caffeine that promotes autophagy; however, as decaffeinated coffee has also proven to induce autophagy in the brain. The antioxidants in coffee are one component of it that promotes autophagy, along with the caffeine. The combination of coffee and the caffeine it contains make regular caffeinated coffee a great food to trigger autophagy in the brain. The caffeine in coffee induces autophagy in the brain, which acts to protect against disorders of the brain such as Alzheimer's or dementia.

- Coffee Cherry

Similarly to the example of coffee above, the actual coffee cherry from which the coffee beans are extracted is also loaded with beneficial components that are great for promoting autophagy in the brain. In addition to the beans themselves and the caffeine and antioxidants they contain, the actual cherry fruit contains many other elements that are beneficial to the brain and brain health.

- Green Tea

Green tea is another beverage that has been found to induce autophagy in the brain. Green tea contains some caffeine, which you now know induces autophagy, thus protecting the brain, but it also contains another antioxidant which is different from that found in coffee. This antioxidant is called EGCG and is known for its positive effects on the brain. EGCG triggers autophagy in brain cells, which also cleans the brain of degeneration and clears toxic cells, which prevents disorders of the brain and keeps the brain functioning as well as possible. The way that green tea triggers autophagy is also beneficial for memory and learning. The benefits of green tea are far-reaching because of and in addition to its effect on autophagy.

- Coconut Oil

Coconut oil is another extremely beneficial food to ingest in order to improve and maintain a healthy brain through autophagy. Coconut oil is beneficial as it increases the number of ketones in the brain, which, as you learned in the previous chapter, is beneficial for autophagy because ketones in the brain induce autophagy by signaling to the brain cells that there are low levels of energy sources.

Coconut oil can be ingested in a number of ways, which is what makes it such a great food for the brain. You can use coconut oil as cooking oil, in place of a cooking spray, as a substitute in baking, in your coffee, in smoothies, and on your skin.

- Ginger

Ginger is known to be healthy for humans for a number of reasons, such as its amazing ability to treat nausea, its pain-relieving properties, and its benefits for reducing inflammation. In addition to this, it contains a compound called 6-shogaol, which has numerous benefits itself, including its ability to induce autophagy. 6-shogaol also has been shown to reduce the risk of developing cancer as it is an anti-tumor agent as it is able to prevent the uncontrolled growth of cells that develops into a tumor. This is not studied to its full capacity yet, but this ability to stop tumor growth could be due to its effects on autophagy.

Ginger can be ingested in a variety of ways as well, such as in a powder form, as a plant in tea, or in cooking both savory and sweet foods. Many Asian dishes incorporate ginger because of its numerous health benefits.

- Galangal

Galangal is very similar to ginger in the way that it looks, which is why it is often referred to as "thai ginger," however it is actually different than ginger in the way that it tastes. Galangal is not the same as ginger in its wide range of health benefits, but it is similar in that is contains an active compound that induces autophagy in the brain. Further, it is able to specifically benefit the cells associated with dopamine, which is a hormone that leads us to feel happy. This means that Galangal could prove to have benefits for treating depression as well, due to its ability to protect these dopamine-associated brain cells through its induction of autophagy.

- Reishi Mushroom

The Reishi Mushroom is a specific type of mushroom that, like ginger, has many bioactive components.

Bioactive means that it has compounds within it that have an effect on biological organisms like humans. When ingested, these bioactive compounds exert their effects on the body, such as inducing autophagy, for example. This Reishi mushroom, in particular, is able to induce autophagy as well as to regulate it. This means that it is able to cause autophagy to occur as well as regulating the amount and duration of it.

The Reishi mushroom is no new discovery, as it has been used in Chinese medicine for thousands of years as a way of improving immune system function, reducing inflammation, and improving the functioning of the brain. All of these areas that the Reishi mushroom has been known to help are also areas that are impacted by autophagy, which can give us insight into the mechanism by which the bioactive compounds in this mushroom operate.

The Reishi mushroom can be used in cooking or taken in a tincture form for a concentrated dose of the bioactive compounds.

- Turmeric

Turmeric is a rather popular spice in the western world today, found in all types of drinks and foods. This is no new discovery either though, as it is found in Indian curries and has been for decades. Turmeric is so powerful as a spice because it is able to induce autophagy in the brain, which protects them from damage as it clears out damaged cells in order for new ones to replace them.

Turmeric can be found in food like curry, in baking, and in many different sorts of drinks such as tea or in turmeric lattes in virtually every coffee shop these days. Turmeric has a very strong yellow-orange hue that is unmistakable.

- Brussels Sprouts, Cabbage, Kale, Broccoli Sprouts

All of these green vegetables have one thing in common- they all contain Sulforaphane. Sulforaphane is a plant chemical that is found naturally in these vegetables. This is an antioxidant that acts in a similar way to turmeric and thus has similar benefits. Sulforaphane, like turmeric, induces autophagy in the brain, which helps to reduce the risk of Alzheimer's, Parkinson's, and dementia, which are all neurodegenerative diseases. *Neurodegenerative* means that the cells in the brain called nerves are damaged and broken down, which leads to cognitive decline like Alzheimer's or physical decline as in Parkinson's. These vegetables can help to treat these diseases by slowing their progression, as they are all diseases that come about over time. There is no cure yet, but the treatment at this stage involves delaying the progression of these diseases.

Sulforaphane can be found in the aforementioned vegetables, but the strongest source is in broccoli sprouts. It can also be taken concentrated in a supplement form.

- Extra Virgin Olive Oil

Olive oil and extra virgin olive oil, in particular, is beneficial to the health of humans because it has positive effects on inflammation. It is able to reduce inflammation in the brain and the body as well as improve brain functioning as it is able to induce autophagy in the brain. Because of this, extra virgin olive oil, like Sulforaphane, is recommended as a treatment to slow the progression of Alzheimer's disease.

Olive oil can be used for cooking, as a dressing, as a dip and even ingested on its own as a dietary supplement.

- Acai Berries, Strawberries and Blueberries

The bioactive compounds in these specific types of berries work in the brain to induce autophagy and reduce inflammation. This leads to the protection of brain cells in this case from *oxidative stress*. Oxidative stress is something that can happen within the brain when there is an imbalance of oxygen, which can cause reduced cognitive functioning. These berries and their induction of autophagy helps to reduce this by keeping the balance of oxygen at a healthy level.

CHAPTER 6

ANTI-INFLAMMATORY RECIPES

In this chapter, we will look at several recipes that will help you to begin your new anti-inflammatory diet. I encourage you to try these recipes and share them with your family so that they can also benefit from the delicious and healthy anti-inflammatory meals that you will be able to make upon reading this chapter.

Zucchini Noodle Pasta

This is a great recipe for anyone who is looking to add more vegetables to their diet without compromising the delicious flavor of foods they love, such as pasta. This dish packs a flavor punch and is great for you in terms of its health benefits.

NUTRITIONAL INFORMATION:

- 1 serving- half of recipe
- Calories: 362
- Carbohydrates: 16g
- Fiber: 9.1g
- Fat: 6.3g
- Protein: 4.6g

10 mins: Preparation time

5 mins: Cook time

15 mins: Total

INGREDIENTS:

- Water- if and as you need it
- Lemon juice- 1 tablespoon
- Zucchini- 3, cut to strips of ¼ inch width
- Garlic- 1 clove
- Avocado-1
- Fresh basil- ½ cup
- Salt and pepper for tasting
- Olive oil- 2 tablespoons

INSTRUCTIONS:

1. In order for you to make this sauce- combine by placing into a food processor, the avocado,

basil leaves, garlic, and lemon juice, and blend this mixture until it becomes smooth.

2. Next, add the extra virgin olive oil and blend again until incorporated.
3. Add some water, 1 Tablespoon at a time just until the sauce becomes fluid but yet still thick in its consistency.
4. Season this sauce with pepper and salt, to taste.
5. To make the Zucchini Noodles if you have never made them before: use a spiral machine or slice them into thin, noodle-shaped strips.
6. Once you have made your noodles, sauté them in a small amount of olive oil on medium to medium-high temperature, until they become softer and a brighter green hue. This will usually take about 4 minutes.
7. Drain out the extra water from the pan, and you are ready to serve.
8. To Serve: Toss your zucchini noodles in the sauce you made and add some parmesan cheese to the top.
9. (you will likely have some sauce for leftovers, depending on how many macros you are looking to take in).

CAPRESE SALAD WITH BEETS AND AVOCADO

NUTRITIONAL INFORMATION:

Serving Size (1/2 recipe)

Calories: 444

Total Carbohydrates: 5g

Fiber: 1g

Net Carbohydrates: 4g

Fat: 38g

Protein: 22g

INGREDIENTS:

- Unsalted almonds, raw and chopped - ¼ cup
- Kale- 100 grams
- Fresh basil, thinly sliced- to garnish
- Minced shallots- 1 tablespoon
- Buffalo mozzarella cheese, sliced- 1 cup
- Beet- 1 small

- Sea salt- ¼ teaspoon
- Balsamic vinegar- 2 tablespoons
- Extra virgin olive oil- 1 tablespoon
- Freshly ground black pepper- as much as desired

INSTRUCTIONS:

1. Preheat the oven to 400 degrees Fahrenheit. Wrap the beet in some foil. Roast the beet in the foil just until it becomes soft enough to put a fork through it, about 1 hour. When the beet is cool enough to handle, peel it, and cut it into about 8 slices.
2. Meanwhile, using a small vessel, whisk to combine the shallots, vinegar, oil, ⅛ teaspoon salt, and ⅛ teaspoon pepper.
3. Arrange your beet, cheese, and kale on two plates and sprinkle with nuts and basil. Sprinkle evenly with the remaining salt and pepper, and drizzle evenly with the vinaigrette.

GRILLED ASPARAGUS

NUTRITIONAL INFORMATION:

Serving: 4 spears of asparagus

Calories: 50 calories

Carbohydrates: 3.5g,

Protein: 4g,

Fat: 2.5g,

Fiber: 1.5g,

5 mins: prep time

10 mins: cook time

15 mins: total time

INGREDIENTS:

- Olive Oil for greasing
- Kosher salt-for tasting
- black pepper- for tasting
- Asparagus, rimmed at the ends-16
- Parmigiano Reggiano, 1 ounce

INSTRUCTIONS:

1. Drizzle your asparagus on a plate with some olive oil and season it as you wish with black pepper and a pinch of salt.
2. Light up your grill onto only light heat.
3. When the grill is hot enough, clean, and then oil the grates before cooking.
4. Place the asparagus onto your warm grill a begin cooking it for a duration of about 6 mins, with the lid on. Continue cooking them on low heat and turn them every couple of minutes so that they don't burn.
5. Slice the parmigiana very thinly and then add this to the hot asparagus.

VEGAN CHANA MASALA

NUTRITIONAL INFORMATION:

Calories: 371

Calories from Fat: 88

Total Fat: 10g

Carbohydrates: 59 grams

Protein: 17 grams

Servings: Makes 4 Servings

INGREDIENTS:

- Olive Oil-1 Tablespoon
- Cayenne Pepper- 1/8 of a tablespoon
- Diced Tomatoes- 28 ounces diced
- Garam Masala- 2 tablespoons
- Jalapeno Pepper- 1
- Onion- 1 diced
- Ginger- 1 tablespoon shaved
- Garlic- 4 cloves minced
- Chickpeas- canned- 28 ounces (be sure to

drain the liquid and rinse them before using them in the recipe)

INSTRUCTIONS:

1. Take a big wok and put the olive oil into it
2. Once heated, add in your onions and sauté them until they are sweating and softened. This will take about 5 minutes.
3. Add in your ginger, jalapeno, and your garlic, and then cook this mixture for another minute
4. Sprinkle in your spices (pepper, salt, coriander, turmeric, garam masala, cumin, cayenne pepper). Then, cook this for another minute. The mixture will become fragrant as you do this.
5. Add your chickpeas and tomatoes into the fragrant mixture in the wok. Let this simmer.
6. Cover the pan and let this simmer for about twenty minutes.
7. After it simmers for the allotted time, give it a taste test and season it if you feel it could be spicier or if it needs more salt. You might want to mix in some more of the garam masala if you want it to be stronger in flavor.
8. Serve and enjoy this meal!

INSTANT POT TORTILLA SOUP

NURITIONAL INFORMATION:

Serving: 1/8 of Recipe

Calories: 390

Total Carbohydrates: 24 Grams

Protein: 24 Grams

INGREDIENTS:

- Boneless, Skinless Chicken Breasts- 2
- Canned or Frozen Corn- 8 ounces
- Black Beans, canned- 16 ounces
- Diced Tomatoes with Jalapenos, canned -16 ounces
- *You can also include your own fresh jalapeno peppers or other chilis to add spice if you wish.
- Crushed Tomatoes, Canned- 16 ounces
- Onion, diced- 1 large
- Garlic Powder- 1 tbsp

- Chicken Broth- 4 cups
- Chili Powder- 2 tsp
- Tortilla Strips- As many as you wish
- Cumin- 2 tsp
- Shredded Cheese, Sour Cream, Cilantro or any other toppings you want to put on to serve it

INSTRUCTIONS:

1. In your Instant Pot, put your beans, the corn, and your Onions and the diced tomatoes (with chilis or add the jalapenos separately at the same time)
2. Then, put in the chicken breasts
3. Sprinkle in the garlic powder, chili powder, and cumin
4. Next, pour in your crushed tomatoes and your chicken broth
5. Turn it on to manual high pressure
6. Cook for 30 minutes at this setting
7. Press Quick Release
8. Take the chicken out of the Instant Pot and shred it into small strips or pieces
9. Put your shredded chicken into the Instant Pot and mix everything together
10. Serve by putting your tortilla chips on top
11. This can be served with any toppings you

wish, such as shredded cheese, sour cream, cilantro for topping, or any other toppings that you would normally put on your tacos!

Avocado Egg Bowls

NUTRITIONAL INFORMATION:

Serving size 130g (One half of recipe)

Calories 215

Fat 18g

Carbohydrates 8g

Fiber 2.6g

Calories from fat 163

Protein 9g

INGREDIENTS:

- Coconut oil- 1 Teaspoon
- Organic, free-range eggs-2
- Salt and pepper- to sprinkle
- Large & ripe avocado- 1

For Garnishing:

- Chopped walnuts, as many as you like
- Balsamic Pearls

- Fresh thyme

INSTRUCTIONS:

1. Slice your avocado in two, then take out the pit and remove enough of the inside so that there is enough space inside to accommodate an entire egg.
2. Cut off a little bit of the bottom of the avocado so that the avocado will sit upright as you place it on a stable surface.
3. Open your eggs and put each of the yolks in a separate bowl or container. Place the egg whites in the same small bowl. Sprinkle some pepper and salt to the whites; according to your personal taste, then mix them well.
4. Melt the coconut oil in a pan that has a lid that fits and put it on med-high.
5. Put in the avocado boats, with the meaty side down on the pan, the skin side up and sauté them for approx. 35 seconds, or when they become darker in color.
6. Turn them over, then add to the spaces inside, almost filling the inside with the whites of the eggs.
7. Then, reduce the temperature and place the lid. Let them sit covered it for approx. 16 to 20 minutes, until the whites are just about fully cooked.

8. Gently add one yolk onto each of the avocados and keep cooking them for 4 to 5 mins, just until they get to the point of cook you want them at.

9. Move the avocados to a dish and add toppings to each of them using the walnuts, the balsamic pearls, or/and thyme.

BUFFALO CHICKEN LETTUCE WRAPS

NUTRITIONAL INFORMATION:

Serves- Makes 3 cups of chicken

Serving Size- 1/2 cup

Fat: 0 grams

Carbohydrates: 5.5 grams

Protein: 24 grams

Sodium: 879 milligrams

Fiber: 12 grams

Sugar: 2 grams

Calories: 148 kcal

INGREDIENTS:

- Boneless, Skinless Chicken Breasts- 3
- Celery stalk, diced- 1
- Onion, diced- One Half

- Garlic, minced- 1 clove
- Chicken Broth, Fat-Free, Low-Sodium- 16 ounces
- Cayenne pepper sauce or other hot sauce- 16 ounces

Wrap Ingredients:

- Lettuce leaves- 6 Large sized leaves
- Carrots, shredded- 1 and ½ Cups
- Celery Stalk, Sliced into small matchstick shapes - 2 large stalks

INSTRUCTIONS:

This recipe can be done using either a slow cooker or an instant pot, whichever you wish to use will work well, but the instructions will be slightly different. Below, you can see both of the recipes for these two options.

1. In your slow cooker, put in the chicken breasts, the celery stalk, the onions, the minced garlic, and the chicken broth.
2. Make sure that your chicken broth is enough to cover the chicken breasts. If not, you can add some water to the broth in order to cover the chicken breasts.
3. Put the lid on and cook this at a high setting for a duration of 4 hours of cooking time, if

using a slow cooker. If using an instant pot, Cover your Instant Pot with the lid and turn it on to its high-pressure setting for 15 minutes. Then, allow it to naturally release.

4. Remove the chicken from the pot.
5. Take out also 1/2 of a cup of broth from the slow cooker and set it aside. You can discard the rest of the broth.
6. Then, shred the chicken using a knife or fork and then put it back into the slow cooker, as well as your reserved one-half cup of broth.
7. Add the hot sauce to the pot as well and then turn the slow cooker setting to "high" and cook this for 30 more minutes. If using an instant pot, add the hot sauce to the pot as well and then turn the Instant Pot to the sauté setting. Sauté for 2 to 3 minutes.
8. While this is cooking, get your lettuce wraps ready. To do this, put ¼ of a cup of carrots, any dressing you wish, and the celery matchsticks into the lettuce wrap.
9. When the chicken is finished, add this to your lettuce wraps, and then they are ready!
10. Wrap up and start eating!

CHAPTER 7

30-DAY MEAL PLAN

In this chapter, you are going to learn how to create your own meal plan. The meal plan provided for you has been created in order to help you begin your journey toward your new lifestyle. By having a meal plan to follow, you will be able to set yourself up for success by making it easier for yourself to follow this new way of eating.

Meal Plan

In the section that follows, you can see a sample one-week meal plan. For the first week, it will be beneficial for you to follow this meal plan specifically. If you are a vegetarian, you can substitute some of the meals for vegetarian-friendly dishes, but several of the dishes in this sample meal plan are vegetarian already.

Sunday

- Breakfast

  Avocado Egg Boats

- Lunch

  Grilled Shrimp Kebabs

- Dinner

  Green Beans and Tofu Stir-Fry

- Snacks and Dessert

  Grilled Asparagus Snack

Monday

- Breakfast

  Breakfast Smoothie

- Lunch

  Chicken Lettuce Wraps

- Dinner

  Cauliflower Kale Soup

- Snacks and Dessert

Green Smoothie Snack

Tuesday

- Breakfast

Greek Yogurt with blueberries

- Lunch

Leftover Cauliflower Kale Soup

- Dinner

Tortilla Soup

- Snacks and Dessert

No dessert (can be switched to any other day or multiple other days)

Wednesday

- Breakfast

Non-Fat yogurt with berries

- Lunch

Turkey breast with roasted broccoli

- Dinner

Vegetarian Chilli

- Snacks and Dessert

Stone Fruit snack- a peach for example

Thursday

- Breakfast

Greens Smoothie

- Lunch

Leftover Vegetarian chili

- Dinner

Fish filet and Salad

- Snacks and Dessert

Greek Yogurt with Berries

Friday

- Breakfast

Overnight Oats

- Lunch

Homemade Turkey and Vegetable soup

- Dinner

Broccoli Beef Stir-Fry

- Snacks and Dessert

Choice of Fruit

Saturday

- Breakfast

  Spinach Scrambled Eggs

- Lunch

  Roasted Brussels Sprouts

- Dinner

  Salmon with a Caprese salad

- Snacks and Dessert

  Berries

How to Create Your Own Meal Plan

For your second, third and fourth weeks, you can choose one of three options;

1. You can stick with the same weekly meal plan if you are a person who likes and appreciates routine, and you have come to enjoy having your meals planned for you like this.
2. You can substitute the meals that you did not enjoy for new ones, taking them from the recipe chapter earlier on in this book, and keep the meals that you did enjoy the same.
3. You can change up the meal plan entirely,

taking them from the recipe chapter at the end of this book if you are a person who likes to change things up and who does not enjoy eating the same meals each week.

With this meal plan, you can substitute anything you wish with the recipes included in this book, or with other recipes that you find which adhere to the guidelines that you have learned in this book. The best thing about it is that you can also take leftovers for lunch at work the next day if you make something for dinner that you just can't get enough of!

Some other foods that you can substitute this meal plan with include the following,

- Lettuce Wraps
- Tortilla Soup
- Grilled Asparagus
- Caprese salad with beets
- And so on…

Or anything else that is anti-inflammatory that you wish to include in your weekly eating plan.

Tips for Success

In this section, I will share with you several tips to help you find success with following your new meal plan, especially during the first few weeks of your new diet plan.

- Meal Preparation

In addition to this, it will be greatly helpful for you if you prepare your meals in advance. When it comes to trying to implement a lifestyle change or a new habit that involves food or dieting, meal prep will be a key to your success. Meal prep is when you prepare meals like your lunch or pieces to your dinner in advance so that you can easily prepare or reheat them later. You can meal prep an entire week's worth of lunches for yourself on the weekend, and all you would have to do in the morning before you leave for work or school is to take one out of the fridge. Then at lunch, you just pop it in the microwave, and you have a delicious and healthy lunch ready for you in under five minutes. You can prepare parts of your dinner in a similar way as well like preparing meat with a marinade the night before or cooking some chicken breast to reheat at dinner time.

- Pay attention to your hunger

It can be hard to tell sometimes when we are really hungry, and when we may be feeling as though food will make us feel better emotionally. Real hunger is when our body needs nutrients or energy and is letting us know that we should replenish our energy soon. This happens when it has been a few hours since our last meal when we wake up in the morning, or after a lot of strenuous activity like a long hike. Our body uses hunger to signal to us that it is in need of more energy and that if it doesn't get it soon, it will begin to use our stored energy as fuel. While there is nothing wrong with our body using its stored fuel, it can be used as a sign to us that we should eat shortly in order to replenish these stores.

Perceived Hunger is when we think we are hungry, but our body doesn't actually require any more energy or for the stores to be replenished. This can be because our brain notices that it is the time of day when we would normally eat, even if we have just eaten a short time before when we are feeling stressed or anxious, and our body isn't sure how to soothe this so we think that food may help. It is important to be aware of this because these are the times when we would most often reach for something convenient and packaged, which is not food that is included within the parameters of the anti-inflammatory diet. Our brains know that we can get comfort and feelings of reward from foods that are high in sugar, salt, and fat, so it will tell you this in the form of cravings.

Before giving in to these cravings, ensure that you are, in fact, experiencing actual hunger, and instead of giving your body the sugary food it craves, reach for one of your pre-prepared meals or snacks instead.

When we feel hungry, there are several questions we can ask ourselves to determine whether we are, in fact, hungry and in need of sustenance, or we are hungry because of an emotional need, boredom, or stress. In order to help you determine this, you can ask yourself the following questions;

1. How hungry am I?

Go within and ask yourself how hungry you are. While you don't want to wait until you are absolutely starving and light-headed to eat, you want to be hungry enough. If you are not quite at a level where you could eat a meal, you probably aren't hungry enough to eat just yet.

2. When did I last have a meal?

We want to ask ourselves this question because if we had a full meal less than 2 or 3 hours ago, it is likely that we are not experiencing actual hunger, but the hunger is coming from something else like an emotional need or boredom.

3. Was there a change in my emotional state just previously?

Sometimes, we will feel the need or the compulsion to eat right after we get some bad news or have an upsetting thought or conversation. Ask yourself if you felt the feeling of hunger directly after one of these occurrences or something that you know to be a trigger for your emotional hunger. If something like this has just happened, you may not have connected them as being related. By taking a minute to recognize this, you can decide that you may not actually be hungry and address the emotional issue instead.

4.   Am I still Hungry Now?

If you feel hungry, try drinking a glass of water. Wait twenty minutes and see if you are still hungry afterward. If you are not, you could have just been hungry because of your emotional state.

5.   Pay attention to your plate composition

It can be hard to know how much to eat and when you have had enough without going to the point where you have eaten too much and feel completely full. This section includes some tips on how much to eat so that you can begin to tell how much the right amount for you is. This guide helps us to determine the protein to carbohydrates to vegetable ratio of each of our meals. We don't want to have a plate that is 80 percent carbohydrates, or that is lacking in vegetables altogether. If we have a properly balanced plate, we will be giving our body everything it needs to function, and this will make it less likely that we will be hungry shortly after a meal, which is when we would be reaching for a snack. By giving our body the right amount of protein and vegetables, especially, this will keep us satisfied for longer, and then a snack will be the last thing on our minds. This helps to take care of one large part of the emotional eating equation- if you are satisfied from your meal for longer, you will be less inclined to eat a snack that is full of ingredients that will increase your body's level of inflammation.

When it comes to protein, we want to make sure we are eating enough of it because this is what keeps us full for longer. Protein takes longer to digest than carbohydrates; therefore, it gives us energy for longer. When it comes to putting protein in your meal, you want the cooked and finished product to be roughly the size of your palm.

If you have ever had a meal or a snack that was largely composed of carbohydrates- especially the extremely processed kind, then you likely felt hungry again shortly after finishing. This is a big reason why meal composition is an important topic to become educated on. In today's societies, many of our meals will be mostly composed of carbohydrates, which is likely why many of us tend to remain hungry after a meal. When you are putting carbohydrates into your meal, you want the finished and cooked product to be about one handful worth.

When it comes to vegetables, many of us eat much less than we should. It is said that vegetables should make up half of your plate if you want to be an extremely healthy eater. What we will say here is that your meal should be composed of an amount of vegetables roughly the size of your fist, at minimum.

When it comes to fats, not all of them are bad. We do not need to omit all fats from our diet as some of them are good fats that can actually help to lower the bad cholesterol and increase the good cholesterol. When we hear about fats and cholesterol, we tend to only hear about the bad kinds, which makes us afraid of fats altogether. When it comes to adding fats to a meal, the rule is that you can have an amount of fat that is equivalent to the size of your thumb.

With these guides that use your own hand as a tool, it accounts for different body sizes and body compositions. As you know, a tall man will need to eat more than a small woman. A tall man, however, will also have a bigger hand. Therefore a bigger fist, palm, and thumb and their plate size will be bigger as well. This is a foolproof tool as this takes away any calorie counting, determining weight and body composition or math needed to figure out the size that your meal should be. This makes it quick and easy and makes it so that anyone can do it anywhere. If you are at a restaurant, it will also help you to determine how much to eat and what you will order. Restaurant meals tend to be the worse culprits for including a disproportionate amount of carbohydrates and little to no vegetables. Keeping this in mind, you may decide to order a side of vegetables and pack up some of the carbohydrates in the meal to take home for lunch the next day.

6.   Eat slowly

When we eat, it takes about twenty minutes for the hormone in our bodies that tells us that we are full to reach our brain. Our stomach signals to our brain that we are hungry and that signal takes about twenty minutes to reach the brain. Thus, we want to make sure that we eat slowly so that we can tell when we are full. If we eat very quickly, by the time we get the signal that we are full, we will have already eaten much more than we may have needed. When you feel like you may be satiated, stop eating and wait for about twenty minutes. You will likely feel full then, but if not, you can always eat a bit more then.

CHAPTER 8

HOW TO STICK TO YOUR NEW DIET

In this chapter, I will share with you some tips for sticking to your diet and making it a habit in your daily life. Your health is important, and sticking to a plan that will improve and maintain your health is very important, as you have seen throughout this book.

To begin, I will define the term *motivation* for you. Motivation is different for every person, in every scenario, but it is possible to reduce this to a single definition for this term. Motivation is something within a person that drives the wish to change something about their life. Motivation, then, comes down to wanting something that you do not have. These desired changes can be internal or external- in a person's environment. Motivation combines with the desire to change in order to make a person take action and steps toward their desired outcomes. Motivation is what helps people accomplish things that they set out to do. Some motivation is triggered by needs, such as the need to sustain your life (eating, sleeping, etc.), and some are triggered by the needs of a psychological nature, such as the need to have a human connection.

Throughout this book, we have revisited the term motivation over and over again in order to help you to ensure the most success possible. By examining your motivations, you will be likely to stay on track. By understanding your motivations for something that you wish to achieve, it helps you to remember why you began and helps you to push through when things become difficult.

In this final chapter of the book, we will discuss the mind-body connection and how this will help you to stay on track. Be prepared for some self-reflection and realization, which is the first step in making any changes in one's life.

How to Make Your New Diet a Habit

In this section, we will look at a variety of ways that

you can begin to make your motivation to continue in the pursuit of your new lifestyle. Making your motivation a daily habit will come down to self-discipline. We are going to look at some ways that you can improve and maintain self-discipline in the face of challenging times.

- Break it up Into Smaller Sections

To strengthen self-discipline, you need to work on instilling a new habit, which can feel very intimidating at first, especially if you are focusing on the entire goal all at once. To avoid this daunting feeling, keep it very simple. Break your bigger goal into smaller doable ones. Instead of trying to accomplish one huge goal all at once or to change all of your habits all at once, focus on doing just one thing consistently and exercise your self-discipline with that one small thing.

For example, if you are somebody that is looking to get into better shape, start by exercising for 10 to 15 minutes per day. Instead of trying to go to the gym for 2 hours every day, which can be very daunting, start with a smaller goal in mind first. By taking baby steps, you can get your mind used to that habit and slowly increase the amount of time that you spend at the gym. Eventually, once you feel like that goal has become a habit, you can then begin to focus on other small goals and keep building up words from there.

- Work On Self-Discipline

Self-discipline is not something that people are born with; rather, it is a learned behavior. Self-discipline is just like any other skill that people may be looking to grow. It requires repetition and lots of daily practice. Similar to going to the gym, the more you work out your muscles, the bigger and stronger they will become. Changes do not happen overnight, instead to strengthen your muscles and to grow them; It will take at least several weeks for a person to be able to see their progress. The effort and focus that training self-discipline requires can be extremely tiring, but it is extremely rewarding in the long run.

- Set Clear Goals for Yourself

In order to continue strengthening your self-discipline, a person must have a clear vision of what goals they are trying to accomplish. They must also have an understanding of what success means to them. If a person doesn't know where they're planning to go or what accomplishing their goals even and Tails, it is easy for them to lose their way or to get sidetracked.

Make sure the goals that you are setting have a clear and concise purpose. For example, don't use goals like "I want to be rich by the next five years." This goal is too broad for it to have a strong meaning. Instead, you should make a goal that is quantifiable like "I am planning on saving $20,000 by the end of this year". Then, when you have a quantifiable goal, you are able to make a plan that makes sense for yourself. In this example, a person can plan to save $2,000 each month for the rest of this year in order to hit their goal of saving $20,000 by the end of it. They can break down these goals even further and figure out where in their budget they can save money or how they can make more money to accomplish that goal.

How to Remain Focused on Your Diet

- Find your motivation or your reason "why"

Everybody's objective will differ slightly and will likely be quite personal to them. Maybe you want to reduce your risk of cancer because it runs in your family. Maybe you have been obese for the majority of your life, and you are trying this as a means of weight loss and health improvement. If you are unsure of your motive or your "why," take some time to look deep within yourself and address the reasons why you are reading this book or the reasons why you feel it is time to make a change in your life. By taking stock of your feelings this will lead you to find your motivation for seeking change.

- Don't underestimate the power of your mind

When it comes to something like changing your eating behaviors or changing your exercise level, the mental game is the biggest part of it. You already know that your body can survive the exercise or the changes in diet. You know that you will not be starving yourself or running yourself into the ground by exercising. You know that your body will likely even be better for having done these things. What all this means is that the part that makes change so difficult is the mental part. As you begin to make changes to your lifestyle, the mindset will play a huge part in how successful you will be.

What you choose to focus on from day to day will determine whether you are having a terrible time, counting down the hours until you can eat, or whether you barely notice those hours going by.

By focusing on what you are depriving yourself of, or on all of the things that you are not doing anymore, you will see everything as a punishment. This will make it very difficult for you to make it through each day of your new lifestyle, as everything will seem like it has been changed and replaced with some type of punishment.

By instead looking at the things that you are giving yourself- like fresh foods, a healthier diet, weight loss, and self-care, and appreciating these things, it will help you to rediscover the positivity in small things, such as how refreshing and nourishing water is for example, which is a fact that we take for granted in places where our water is clean and drinkable. You will be able to appreciate the fresh foods that have been grown by farmers in order to nourish your precious body. You will also appreciate your food that much more when you have selected it because of the benefits that it will give your body. By viewing your day through the lens of appreciation instead of deprivation, you will have a much easier time with your fast, and this will lead you to stay motivated. Then, motivation will eventually become an automatic thought process instead of a conscious decision that you need to make each day.

- Acknowledge your feelings

When emotions come up during the beginning stages of your new diet, it is important to know what to do with them. The first step is to acknowledge them. By acknowledging these emotions, you can tap into them and examine them in more depth. The next step is to write them down. This can be a very quick note of how you are feeling or what you are finding the most challenging part of this new diet to be for you. By writing down these feelings, you are processing this emotion, and you are able to address it instead of pushing it away. When we push our emotions away, they do not really go away; they just go dormant for a short period of time only to come up later. This can result in feelings of discomfort and the urge to put your diet aside entirely. By instead addressing them, you can examine what is going on inside of you and deal with it in the moment so that it does not come up later on and throw you off of your new diet plan.

Tips for Staying on Track

- Write down your goals

Whatever your objective, writing it down will help to solidify it and make it more real. By having it written down on paper, you will have put your reason for doing all of this out into the universe, and it will make you feel as if there is no going back now. This will keep you motivated when times get tough. You can revisit that paper anytime you need a reminder of why you are taking on such a challenge. Seeing that paper will remind you of why it is all worth it. When you are wondering why on earth you decided to put yourself through this as you begin to incorporate new behaviors into your daily routine, you can look back on your reason for beginning in the first place (that you wrote down), and it will re-inspire you to continue. This will enable you to keep going even when you feel as though it is difficult, and this is what will lead to lasting changes. When it comes to mindset, being aware of your motivation is extremely beneficial.

- Expect challenges, and keep going

By expecting that there will be some uncomfortable side-effects such as cravings or irritability, you can greet them with the feeling of having expected them, rather than the feeling of dread that you are feeling this way. If you are not surprised that you will feel a little bit uncomfortable while your body adapts to this new lifestyle, you will be able to greet this uncomfortability rather than fight it, which will make you much more comfortable, as fighting it will not change the reality of it.

It is important to recognize when taking on a new diet or a new lifestyle that this is a choice you are making for your health and your body (or whatever specific objective you have). You must recognize that this is a choice you are consciously making and that you have decided to go through the challenges and sometimes uncomfortable moments in order to receive the benefits later. If you lose sight of the fact that this is a choice you are making, you may begin to feel like a victim or that the universe is punishing you. This victim mindset will only make things harder for you. By taking responsibility for your decision to change your life, you will not allow yourself to slip into this negative mindset and will instead feel confident and in control of your decision. This is another perspective that will help you to view things through the lens of appreciation rather than deprivation, as I described above.

- Don't wait for motivation

People often have the wrong mindset where they think that they need to feel fully motivated before they start working on a task/job. This mindset is unrealistic. People's motivation often does not arrive until they have started that task and are beginning to see progress. When people see progress, they start to see the fruits to their labor, and they become even more motivated to keep working until they have completed their task. You might be wondering what about the motivation that is needed in order to start working altogether? The answer to this is that a person needs to have a good understanding of the 'why' and the vision of that particular job. Before you even begin working on it, you should know what the benefits are going to be. You would be surprised at how many people waste a lot of time doing work that actually does not need to be completed. Moreover, people should be using prioritization in order to get the most urgent and important work out of the way first. By understanding the benefits of completing a task or job, you will fully be able to estimate its importance. In terms of smaller tasks/jobs, simply understanding what the benefits are of completing that task should be enough for motivation. For larger tasks and jobs, it is important that you have a way to measure your progress so you can further gain motivation and confidence from your work.

One main reason that people put off doing the work that they need to do is that they subconsciously find that their work is too overwhelming for them. Start by just breaking down whatever that task is into littler parts and then focus on one at a time. If you find yourself still wanting to procrastinate after you've already broken it down, then break it down even more. You will eventually get to a point where the task that you need to do is so easy that you would feel very badly about yourself if you didn't just do it. If you are struggling with motivation, this is a great way to cope, as it can help you to put one foot in front of the other and get started so that your motivation will begin to grow as you begin to see results.

- Maintain a "Growth Mindset"

By expecting that there will be some uncomfortable side-effects like hunger and irritability, you can greet them with the feeling of "Oh hello, I have been expecting you." Rather than "Oh no, I am feeling so terrible, what is going on?" If you are not surprised that you will feel a little bit uncomfortable while your body adapts to your fast, you will be able to greet it rather than fight it, which will make you much more comfortable with it all.

It is important to recognize when fasting, that this is a choice you are making for your health, your body, or whatever specific objective you have. You must recognize that this is a choice you are consciously making and that you have decided to go through these times of fasting in order to later receive the benefits. If you lose sight of the fact that this is a choice you are making, you may begin to feel like a victim or like the universe is punishing you. This victim mindset will only make things harder for you. By taking responsibility for your decision to fast, you will not allow yourself to slip into this negative mindset and will instead feel confident and in control of your decision. This will help you to view things through the lens of appreciation rather than deprivation like I outlined above.

Success depends on whether or not a person has a growth mindset. A fixed mindset is when a person believes that their intelligence and skills are a fixed trait. They have what they have, and that's it. This makes the person highly concerned with what skills and intelligence they currently have, and they do not focus on what they can gain. Therefore, their activities are limited to the capacity that they think they have. However, those with growth mindsets understand that skills and intelligence is something that can be developed and learned throughout the course of their life. This can be done through education, training, or simply just even passion. They understand that their brain is a muscle that can be 'worked out' to grow stronger.

Knowing this, it is important that you employ a growth mindset. Every single skill you have, and anything that you wish to try or to improve upon can be ameliorated by putting in the effort to see it from a growth mindset. This is the mindset for success when it comes to life in general, but especially when it comes to changing something about your lifestyle-like beginning an intermittent fasting regimen.

Think about what mindset you have right now. If you already have a growth mindset, you simply need to continue practicing it while being proactive about avoiding obstacles and overcoming failures. If you think you are someone with a fixed mindset, change it right now. Believe me when I tell you that intelligence and skills can be improved upon with time and hard work. If you don't believe me, just try it. Pick a random skill; this could be knitting, programming, jogging, or anything that can be learned. Set goals for yourself and begin learning something new. If you are able to take something that you have zero skill in and become proficient in it, you have just proved to yourself that growth mindsets are real and fixed mindsets only hold you back from success.

CONCLUSION

O nce again, I would like to congratulate you on taking the first step towards building a healthier you!

As you now know, inflammation is a process within the body that is meant to help you maintain a healthy body free of disease or damage. The problem comes about, however, when this inflammation does not go away and becomes a chronic problem in your body. When this happens, a person can be left with many negative side-effects, including chronic pain or a variety of different inflammation-related diseases, which you now understand in much more depth than you did at the beginning of this book.

With The World Health Organization telling us that diseases related to chronic inflammation are the number one cause of death in the entire world, this has raised red flags for many people and caused them to look at their lifestyles and their diets from a critical perspective. I hope that this book has helped you to do that and that it has helped you to figure out what you can begin to do in order to change this trajectory of your health and your life. You now understand that you have a large part to play in preventing these diseases within your own body before they begin.

The WHO also stated that the prevalence of chronic inflammatory diseases is projected to increase greatly over the next thirty years, which has gotten many people concerned about the health of their children and their grandchildren. The great thing is that by changing your diet and your lifestyle, you can set a great example for your children and their children so that they can grow up healthily and free of inflammatory disease. With statistics such as these, there has never been a better time to share this book with others and to begin taking your health into your own hands by changing your diet.

Written in an easy to digest manner, this book aims to help you to break the cycle of inflammatory disease and prevent yourself from becoming a statistic! Begin changing your diet today, and you will start to feel better from now on.